Weight Stability

How the Body Regulates Energy Balance, Storage, and Long-Term Change

Nathan Reed

PERENNIAL PUBLISHING

Published by Perennial Publishing

Paperback ISBN: 978-1-971996-45-5
Hardcover ISBN: 978-1-971996-46-2
E-book ISBN: 978-1-971996-47-9

Contents

Weight as a Delayed System Output

Weight is unusually visible compared with most internal metabolic processes. It can be measured quickly, repeated often, and compared across time with little effort. The number is simple enough to remember and precise enough to appear definitive. Because it is visible, it often carries more interpretive weight than the system that produces it. The number appears to explain itself.

This creates a specific kind of interpretive risk. A number can be accurate while still being incomplete. It can represent a real state at a given moment while failing to describe how that state was produced or what it represents across time. Visibility makes the signal accessible, but accessibility does not guarantee clarity. The number is easy to obtain, but not inherently easy to understand.

In many contexts, weight becomes more than a measurement. It is treated as a target to reach, a verdict to interpret, or a score to react to. This framing places the number at the center of the system, as though it were the primary variable to be managed. It encourages the assumption that changes in behavior should translate directly and immediately into changes in the visible output. When that translation is not clean, the number appears inconsistent or difficult to explain.

The limitation of this framing is structural rather than cultural. Treating weight as a target or verdict separates it from the system that produces it. It places emphasis on the output while reducing attention to the processes that generate that output across time. The number becomes primary, and the system becomes secondary. Interpretation then relies on the assumption that the number reflects immediate conditions rather than accumulated ones.

This book begins from a different position.

Weight is not the system itself. It is one output produced by the system.

That distinction shifts the interpretive frame without dismissing the number. Weight remains visible and measurable, but it is repositioned as a signal rather than a command point. It reflects the cumulative result of many interacting processes: intake, expenditure, storage, release, fluid balance, hormonal coordination, appetite, glucose handling, recovery state, adaptation, compensation, and time. These processes operate continuously, often without direct visibility, and their interaction produces the output that appears on the scale.

The number is therefore real, but incomplete. It represents the visible surface of a deeper structure. It shows that the system has produced an outcome, but it does not, on its own, explain how that outcome came to be.

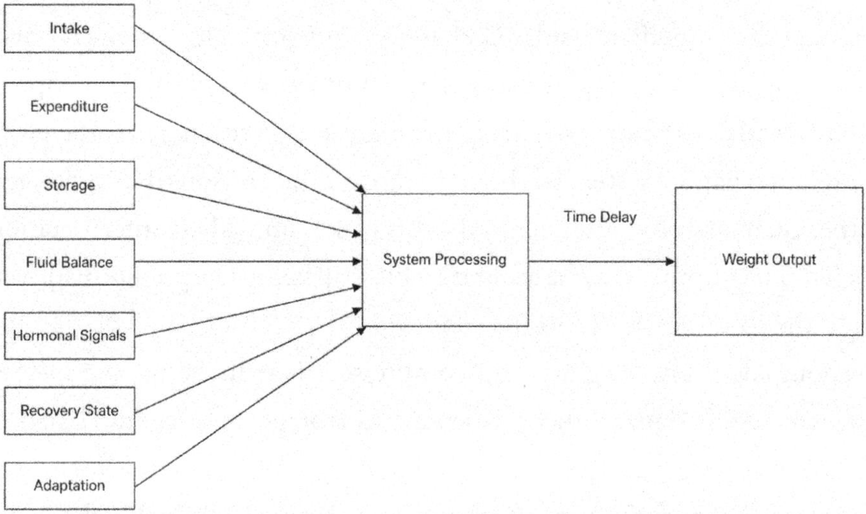

[Figure 1: Weight as a Delayed System Output]

The figure represents weight as the visible endpoint of a series of upstream processes. Energy enters the system through intake. It is distributed, stored, released, and used according to current conditions. Hormonal signals coordinate how energy is routed. Fluid balance shifts in response to intake, sodium, recovery, and stress. Adaptation alters how the system responds to repeated conditions. Compensation adjusts variables when one part of the system changes. Across time, these processes accumulate into a visible output. The number on the scale reflects that accumulation. It does not operate as the central control point within it.

Understanding weight as an output also requires understanding that it is delayed. The number observed at a given moment does not belong entirely to that moment. It reflects prior conditions—patterns of intake, energy use, storage and release, recovery demands, sleep, stress, and hormonal coordination that have been unfolding over time. The visible reading is therefore connected to a timeline, not to a single event.

This delay is central to interpretation. A change in input does not produce an immediate, isolated change in output. The system receives input, processes it, distributes energy, buffers variation, and adjusts internal variables before producing a visible result. A reading may therefore represent what the system has been doing over the previous days or longer, rather than what has just occurred. This makes immediate interpretation fragile. The number may be accurate while still being temporally displaced from the conditions that produced it.

Alongside delay, weight is also compressed. It reduces many processes into one visible signal. Intake, expenditure, storage, release, fluid balance, glycogen levels, digestive contents, recovery demands, and hormonal signaling all contribute to the final number. Compression makes the signal useful because it provides a visible output of an otherwise complex system. But compression also removes context. Different internal conditions can produce the same visible number, and similar system patterns can produce different numbers under different circumstances.

This dual property—visibility combined with compression—explains why weight is both informative and easy to misinterpret. It contains real information about the system, but it does not carry enough detail to stand alone as an explanation. The number must be read in relation to the processes that produce it, rather than in isolation.

The concept of stability emerges from this structure. Stability does not refer to a fixed number or the absence of change. It refers to the coherence of the system across time—the relationship between conditions and the output they produce. When the system's behavior is relatively stable, the output becomes more interpretable. When conditions vary unpredictably, interpretation becomes more difficult, even if the number itself appears simple.

Beginning with stability rather than control allows the system to remain visible. Control, as a starting frame, focuses attention on the output and assumes that it can be directed immediately. Stability focuses attention on the conditions that shape the output. It acknowledges that the system operates through regulation, delay, variability, and adaptation. It does not eliminate the possibility of influencing outcomes, but it changes the order of interpretation. Understanding the system precedes attempts to direct it.

This distinction becomes important when considering how weight behaves over time. The number does not move in a clean or linear manner. It can fluctuate from day to day due to fluid shifts, glycogen changes, digestion, recovery demands, sodium intake, and stress. It can remain stable for a period while internal variables are still adjusting. It can change gradually as small mismatches accumulate. It can lag behind underlying changes, appearing static while the system is shifting, or moving while underlying conditions have already stabilized.

These patterns do not represent inconsistency in the system. They reflect the nature of the processes producing the output. Variability introduces short-term noise. Delay separates input from visibility. Adaptation changes how the system responds over time. Compensation alters variables when conditions shift. Storage and release buffer energy across periods of availability and demand. The output is the result of all of these processes interacting across time.

This book does not attempt to simplify these processes into a single explanatory variable. It does not treat weight as a direct reflection of any one factor. Instead, it treats weight as a signal produced by the interaction of many factors. The purpose is not to reduce the system to the number, but to place the number back inside the system that produces it.

For that reason, this is not a book about diets, calorie targets, or behavioral prescriptions. It does not provide instructions for how to change the number. It does not offer protocols for eating, fasting, exercise, or tracking. It does not present weight as a problem to be solved or a target to be reached. Its focus is narrower and more foundational: to explain how weight becomes visible, why it changes, why it sometimes does not change, and why interpretation requires time and context.

The chapters that follow will examine the system through different mechanisms. Some will focus on how weight is produced as an output. Others will examine why the output is delayed or variable. Others will explore how intake, expenditure, storage, hormonal coordination, appetite, adaptation, and compensation interact. Later sections will connect weight to glucose, fasting, and metabolic flexibility, and will develop how trend and consistency affect interpretation. The goal is not to fragment the system into parts, but to make its structure more visible.

The central movement of the book is interpretive. It shifts weight from being treated as an immediate explanation to being understood as delayed evidence of system behavior. That shift does not remove the number's importance. It changes how its importance is understood. The number becomes more useful when it is read as part of a pattern rather than as a standalone event.

This interpretive model also reduces the need for immediate conclusions. A single reading does not need to explain the system. A short period does not need to reveal direction. Variation does not need to be resolved into meaning at once. The system can be observed across time, allowing patterns to emerge from accumulation rather than from isolated points.

Weight remains a real and relevant signal within this model. It reflects the system's behavior in a way that is visible and repeatable. But its meaning depends on how it is interpreted. When the number is treated as the system, interpretation becomes narrow and reactive. When the number is treated as an output of the system, interpretation becomes broader and more stable.

The introduction therefore establishes a single distinction that will carry through the rest of the book:

A visible number is not the same as an immediate explanation.

Output Mechanism

Weight presents itself as a simple signal. A scale produces a single number, and that number appears to summarize the body in a way that feels immediate and complete. It is visible, repeatable, and easily compared across moments. This apparent clarity creates the impression that the body has expressed its condition directly, without ambiguity. The number seems to explain itself.

This is where interpretation begins to narrow too quickly. Visibility is often mistaken for explanation. A value that can be read instantly is assumed to represent a stable and self-contained truth, rather than a compressed result of ongoing processes. The simplicity of the output masks the complexity of what produced it. The scale does not show how the number formed. It shows only that a number exists.

What appears as a single value is the endpoint of multiple interacting processes operating across time. Body weight is not composed of one thing. It includes water distributed across compartments, glycogen stored and depleted in response to intake and demand, digestive contents moving through the gastrointestinal system, structural tissue, and stored energy. Each of these components changes at different rates and in response to different signals. Some shift over hours, others over days, and some over much longer periods.

These components are not independent. They are regulated through coordinated systems that respond to intake, expenditure, hormonal signaling, appetite, recovery state, stress load, and adaptation. Energy enters the system through intake, but how that energy is processed depends on signaling pathways that determine whether it is used immediately, stored, or redistributed. Expenditure reflects both baseline physiological activity and variable demands, but it is also shaped by adaptive responses that alter efficiency over time. Storage is not static; it expands and contracts in relation to these interacting forces.

Fluid balance adds another layer of variability. Changes in sodium handling, stress signaling, inflammation, and hormonal regulation can shift fluid distribution without altering stored energy. Glycogen storage binds water in predictable ratios, meaning that shifts in carbohydrate availability and utilization can produce measurable changes in weight independent of long-term storage. Digestive contents introduce further short-term variation as material enters, moves through, and exits the system. These changes occur continuously, often without direct awareness, yet they contribute to the number that appears on the scale.

Hormonal signaling coordinates these processes. Signals associated with energy availability, stress, and recovery influence how substrates are partitioned, how much energy is expended, and how storage is regulated. Appetite emerges from these same signaling networks, reflecting internal conditions rather than operating as an isolated driver. Recovery state influences how the system allocates resources, with insufficient recovery altering signaling patterns in ways that can shift both expenditure and storage. Stress load interacts with these systems, modifying fluid balance, energy allocation, and signaling precision.

Time integrates all of these processes. Weight is not a momentary expression of a single input. It is the result of accumulated interactions across hours, days, and longer intervals. Some changes appear quickly because certain components respond rapidly. Others emerge slowly because they depend on repeated patterns of input and adaptation. The number on the scale reflects this layering, even though it presents itself as a single, immediate value.

Because the output is compressed, it does not reveal which process has changed. A shift in the number does not specify whether the change came from fluid redistribution, glycogen depletion, digestive variation, altered intake, changes in expenditure, or longer-term storage dynamics. Multiple processes can move in different directions at the same time, with the visible number representing their combined effect. The scale cannot distinguish among these contributions. It reports the result, not the composition.

This compression creates a common interpretive error. When the number is treated as the primary object of attention, it is assumed to be directly responsive to isolated actions or short-term changes. Movement in the output is then interpreted as immediate feedback on those actions. When the number increases, it can be read as a negative outcome; when it decreases, it can be read as a positive one. This interpretation assumes a direct and immediate relationship between action and output, as though the system operates in a simple, linear manner.

The system does not behave that way. Short-term weight movement often reflects fast-changing components such as fluid balance, glycogen levels, and digestive contents. These components can shift substantially without representing changes in longer-term storage. A reduction in glycogen stores, for example, reduces associated water content, producing a visible decrease in weight. Replenishment restores both glycogen and water, increasing weight again. These changes are real, but they do not indicate structural shifts in stored energy. They reflect the dynamics of fuel availability and fluid regulation.

Stress and inflammation can also alter fluid retention, producing increases in weight that are unrelated to energy storage. Changes in intake timing or composition can affect digestive contents, shifting the number without altering underlying tissue. Even within energy balance, the system can redistribute substrates in ways that do not immediately translate into changes in total mass. The visible number moves, but the meaning of that movement depends on the processes that produced it.

When the output is treated as a lever, these distinctions are lost. The number is assumed to be something that can be directly operated, rather than something that emerges from system behavior. This leads to misinterpretation. Normal fluctuation can be mistaken for instability. Delayed responses can be interpreted as absence of change. Short-term decreases can be taken as evidence of lasting shifts, while short-term increases can be seen as reversals. The interpretation becomes detached from the mechanisms that generate the output.

The underlying issue is not the presence of the number, but the way it is used. Weight is often treated as though it contains its own explanation. In reality, it is a compressed signal that requires context to be understood. Without that context, the number is read in isolation, and isolation removes the system from the interpretation. Once the system is removed, the output is left to carry meaning it cannot support on its own.

Understanding weight as a system output restores that context. The number on the scale becomes a visible signal that reflects the combined activity of multiple processes across time. It is downstream of intake, expenditure, storage, signaling, recovery, and adaptation. Each of these processes contributes to the result, but none is fully represented in isolation within the number itself. The output is a convergence point, not a control point.

This distinction changes how the signal is interpreted. Instead of asking what the number should be, the focus shifts to what the number represents. A change in weight becomes evidence that the system has produced a different result, not a directive to act on the number directly. Interpretation moves upstream, toward the processes that generate the output. The question is no longer how to move the number, but how the system has behaved to produce it.

Across longer intervals, patterns begin to emerge from this perspective. While short-term movement can reflect rapidly changing components, longer-term trends reflect accumulated system behavior. Repeated interactions among intake, expenditure, signaling, and adaptation shape these patterns over time. The output integrates these interactions, making it possible to observe directional change when viewed across appropriate timeframes. Even then, the number remains a result rather than a cause. It reflects what has occurred within the system, not what should be imposed upon it.

The scale does not indicate which variable is responsible for a change, nor does it reveal the sequence of events that produced it. It cannot show how intake interacted with expenditure, how signaling influenced storage, or how recovery state modified allocation. It compresses all of this into a single value. That compression is useful for visibility, but it requires interpretation that accounts for what has been compressed.

The relationship between the visible output and the underlying system can be understood as a narrowing process. Multiple inputs—each with its own dynamics, timing, and constraints—converge into one measurable result. The complexity does not disappear simply because it has been expressed as a number. That is why the number alone cannot serve as a complete explanation.

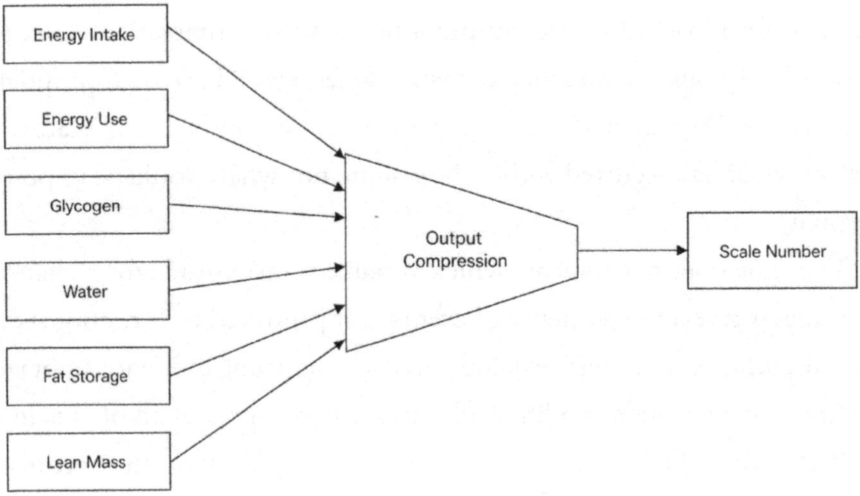

[Figure 2: Multiple Inputs Compress Into One Number]

The figure represents what the scale cannot display: the convergence of multiple upstream processes into a single visible output. Each input—intake, expenditure, storage, fluid balance, signaling, recovery, stress, and adaptation—contributes to the final value. The scale reports the convergence, not the individual contributions.

Once weight is understood in this way, its role changes. It remains visible, but its meaning is reframed. The number is no longer treated as a standalone measure of state. It becomes a piece of evidence within a larger system. It indicates that the system has produced a result, but it does not specify how or why without additional context.

This reframing prepares the ground for further distinctions. If weight is an output, then its behavior across time will reflect the properties of the system that produces it. Delays between input and output, variability in short-term movement, and gradual shifts in longer-term patterns all follow from the fact that multiple processes interact and adapt over time. The output cannot move independently of these processes. It inherits their timing, their constraints, and their dynamics.

Weight becomes useful when it is interpreted with this structure in mind. It is neither dismissed nor elevated beyond its function. It is recognized as a downstream signal that reflects system behavior. The scale provides a value, but the system provides the explanation.

The central correction follows from this: weight is not directly operated. The system produces it. Understanding this distinction shifts interpretation away from the number itself and toward the processes that generate it. When the output is no longer mistaken for the system, the signal it provides can be read in alignment with the mechanisms that shape it.

Lag Mechanism

The number on the scale does not originate at the moment it is read. It arrives after a sequence of internal processes that have already been in motion. What appears as a current measurement is often the visible consequence of prior conditions—intake patterns that have already been processed, expenditure that has already occurred, glycogen that has already been stored or depleted, fluid that has already shifted, and signals that have already influenced allocation and regulation. The scale presents a value in real time, but the system that produces that value operates across time.

This creates a separation between behavior and visible output. The body does not translate each input directly into an immediate change in weight. Instead, inputs move through processes that store, release, buffer, and redistribute energy and mass before any visible expression appears. Internal adjustment precedes external visibility. The scale therefore reflects what the system has already processed, not simply what has just occurred.

This delay is not an error in measurement. It is a property of the system. The body is structured around continuity rather than instant response. Energy entering the system is not immediately expressed as stored mass or reduced mass. It is integrated into existing conditions, directed through signaling pathways, and distributed according to current needs and constraints. Expenditure does not produce an immediate subtraction from visible weight because it draws from available substrates that are themselves regulated and replenished across time. Storage is not instantaneous, and release is not immediate. Each process unfolds with its own timing, influenced by prior states and ongoing regulation.

As a result, the scale rarely reports only current behavior. It reflects a blend of recent and earlier conditions, layered together through ongoing system activity. A change in intake today may not be fully represented in the next visible measurement because other processes—fluid regulation, glycogen dynamics, digestive movement, and prior storage patterns—continue to shape the output. Similarly, a shift in expenditure or recovery state may influence internal allocation before it becomes visible externally. The output lags behind the processes that generate it.

Short-term weight movement is therefore often dominated by components that change quickly. Glycogen is one of the most responsive. Stored glycogen binds water, and changes in glycogen levels alter fluid retention in proportion to those changes. When glycogen is depleted, associated water is released, reducing weight. When glycogen is replenished, water is retained again, increasing weight. These shifts can occur over short intervals and can produce noticeable changes in the scale reading. They are real expressions of system activity, but they do not represent structural changes in stored energy. They reflect fuel availability and fluid coupling.

Fluid regulation extends beyond glycogen. Hormonal signaling related to stress, recovery, and electrolyte balance can alter how fluid is retained or released across compartments. Changes in stress load, sleep quality, or inflammatory signaling can shift fluid distribution, increasing or decreasing visible weight without corresponding changes in long-term storage. These adjustments are part of the system's regulatory response, maintaining internal stability under varying conditions. The scale captures the result of these adjustments, but it does not identify their origin.

Digestive contents introduce another layer of short-term variation. The presence of food within the gastrointestinal system contributes to total mass until it is processed and eliminated. Timing of intake, composition of meals, and transit dynamics can all influence how much material is present at any given time. These variations can shift the number on the scale independently of changes in stored energy. They are transient but measurable, and they contribute to the overall variability of short-term readings.

Inflammation and recovery state further complicate the relationship between behavior and visible output. Tissue stress, whether from physical exertion, illness, or other sources, can lead to localized or systemic inflammatory responses. These responses often involve fluid retention as part of the repair process. Increased fluid can elevate weight temporarily, even as the underlying processes are directed toward restoration. Recovery state influences how resources are allocated, and shifts in that allocation can alter fluid balance and substrate use before any longer-term pattern becomes visible.

These fast-changing components—glycogen, fluid, digestion, and inflammation—can mask or exaggerate slower changes related to storage and release of energy. A reduction in stored energy may be temporarily concealed by increased fluid retention. An increase in stored energy may be obscured by concurrent glycogen depletion. The visible number reflects the combined effect, not the individual contributions. Because these components operate on different timescales, the output can appear inconsistent when viewed over short intervals.

This interaction between fast and slow processes creates the experience of lag. Internal adjustments occur continuously, but their visible expression is filtered through layers of buffering and redistribution. The system absorbs variation, integrates inputs, and only gradually shifts the output in a way that reflects accumulated change. The scale therefore reports delayed consequences rather than immediate reactions.

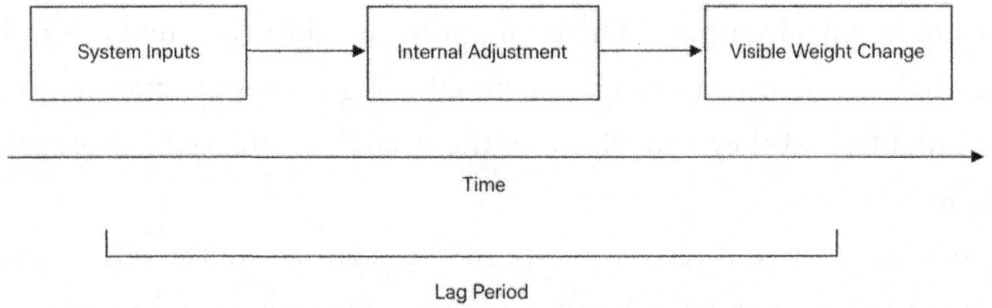

[Figure 3: Lag Between Behavior and Visible Change]

The figure represents this delay as a sequence: inputs enter the system, internal adjustment occurs through storage, release, buffering, and redistribution, and visible weight change emerges after a lag period. The gap between input and output is not empty; it is occupied by coordinated processes that determine how and when change becomes visible.

Understanding this delay clarifies why isolated readings carry limited explanatory power. A single measurement reflects a convergence of processes at a particular moment, shaped by both recent and prior conditions. Without context, it is not possible to determine which processes are responsible for the observed value. Short-term movement can be driven by transient factors that do not indicate longer-term direction. Stability in the output can occur even when underlying processes are shifting, if those shifts are buffered or offset by other changes.

Over longer intervals, patterns begin to emerge that are less influenced by short-term variability. Repeated conditions—consistent intake patterns, sustained expenditure levels, stable recovery states, and ongoing signaling environments—accumulate their effects over time. As these effects accumulate, the influence of transient fluctuations diminishes relative to the broader pattern. The output begins to reflect directional change more clearly, not because the system has become simpler, but because the signal is integrated across enough time to reduce noise from short-term variation.

This does not eliminate variability. Even within longer patterns, fluctuations continue to occur as part of normal system behavior. Fluid shifts, glycogen changes, and digestive variation do not disappear. They continue to contribute to the output, but their relative impact becomes easier to interpret when viewed within a broader temporal context. The pattern provides structure that individual readings cannot.

Expecting the scale to provide immediate confirmation or rejection of recent behavior conflicts with this structure. When the output is interpreted as a real-time indicator, any delay is perceived as inconsistency or failure. A pattern that is stable at the level of system behavior can appear unresponsive because the visible output has not yet adjusted. Conversely, a short-term decrease driven by fluid or glycogen can be interpreted as meaningful change, even though it may not reflect a sustained shift in stored energy. A temporary increase related to inflammation or digestion can be read as reversal, despite being part of normal system fluctuation.

These interpretations arise from a mismatch between expectation and system behavior. The expectation assumes that inputs produce immediate outputs, while the system operates through delayed integration. The scale is then asked to function as a control panel, providing instant feedback on each action. When it does not perform this role, the discrepancy is attributed to inconsistency in the signal rather than to the timing properties of the system.

Lag does not make the signal unreliable. It defines how the signal should be read. A delayed output still contains information, but that information corresponds to prior conditions rather than only current ones. Interpreting the signal requires aligning its timing with the processes that produce it. When the delay is recognized, the apparent inconsistency of short-term readings becomes understandable as the interaction of multiple processes operating on different timescales.

This perspective maintains the usefulness of the scale without assigning it a role it cannot fulfill. The number remains a visible expression of system behavior, but its timing is understood as part of that behavior. The output is not expected to move in direct proportion to each input, nor to reflect each change immediately. It is expected to integrate inputs over time and to express their combined effects after internal adjustment has occurred.

The distinction between immediate input and delayed output also prepares the ground for understanding longer-term dynamics. If weight reflects accumulated system behavior, then changes in pattern—whether stable, variable, or shifting—will appear in the output with corresponding delays. Periods of stability may persist despite underlying change, followed by gradual shifts as the accumulated effects become visible. Variability may increase when fast-changing components dominate, and decrease when conditions stabilize. These patterns are not anomalies; they are expressions of the system's timing and structure.

The scale therefore functions as a delayed signal of prior conditions. It reports what the system has already processed, not what has just occurred. Recognizing this removes the expectation of immediate confirmation and replaces it with an understanding of temporal integration.

The central distinction follows: the scale often reports delayed consequences, not real-time control. This is not a limitation to be corrected. It is a defining characteristic of how the system operates. Weight does not contradict system behavior when it fails to respond immediately. It reflects that behavior unfolding across time.

When the timing of the signal is understood, the apparent gap between action and result becomes part of the explanation rather than a source of confusion. The scale no longer serves as an immediate validator of individual moments. It becomes a record of integrated system activity, arriving after the processes that produce it have had time to unfold.

Variability Mechanism

Daily weight movement presents itself with a level of precision that invites interpretation. The number is specific, measurable, and easily compared to prior readings. It can be written down, remembered, and tracked across time. This visibility creates a sense that the signal is complete, that the body has expressed something definitive about its current state. When the number changes, the change appears concrete. It feels as though something meaningful has occurred and that the scale has captured it clearly.

This sense of clarity is not entirely misplaced. The number does reflect a real measurement. It represents total mass at a given moment. What creates confusion is not the presence of the signal, but the assumption that the signal explains itself. The scale does not isolate a single biological process. It does not distinguish among the components that make up total mass. It reports a compressed result, and that compression gives the appearance of simplicity while concealing the complexity that produced it.

Total mass is not a singular entity. It is a composite of multiple components that move according to different rules and on different timescales. Water is distributed across compartments and can shift rapidly in response to changes in sodium balance, hormonal signaling, and stress load. Glycogen is stored and depleted in relation to energy availability and demand, carrying associated water with it. Digestive contents enter, move through, and exit the gastrointestinal system, contributing to measurable mass while they are present. Stored energy changes more slowly, reflecting accumulated conditions over time rather than immediate inputs. Lean tissue responds to longer-term signals related to recovery, stress, and use. Inflammation and tissue repair can temporarily increase fluid retention, altering mass without representing an expansion of stored energy.

The scale compresses all of these into a single number. It does not indicate which component has changed or how much each component has contributed. A visible shift in weight may reflect a redistribution of water, a change in glycogen storage, the presence or absence of digestive contents, or a longer-term change in stored energy. The number itself does not differentiate among these possibilities. It shows that total mass is different. It does not explain why.

Because the output is mixed, daily fluctuation is expected. The system is not static. It is continuously adjusting to intake, expenditure, signaling, recovery, and environmental conditions. These adjustments involve changes in fluid balance, substrate storage, digestion, and repair processes. Each of these contributes to the measured value. When one or more of these components shifts, the number moves.

Sodium and fluid balance provide one of the most immediate sources of variability. Sodium influences how water is retained and distributed across intracellular and extracellular compartments. Changes in sodium exposure, stress signaling, and hormonal regulation can alter this distribution. The resulting shifts in fluid can increase or decrease measured mass without reflecting a change in long-term energy storage. Hydration status also plays a direct role. Water intake, loss through perspiration, and redistribution within the body all influence the number that appears on the scale.

Glycogen introduces another layer of short-term movement through its relationship with water. Glycogen is stored alongside water, and changes in glycogen availability are accompanied by proportional changes in fluid retention. When glycogen stores are reduced, water is released. When glycogen stores are replenished, water is retained again. These changes can produce noticeable shifts in weight over short intervals. They reflect the system's management of fuel availability and hydration, not a direct indication of fat gain or fat loss.

Digestive contents add further variability. Food and fluid consumed throughout the day contribute to total mass until they are processed and eliminated. The timing of intake, the composition of meals, and the rate of gastrointestinal transit all influence how much material is present at any given time. This means that two readings taken under different digestive conditions can differ even if underlying storage has not changed.

Soreness and tissue repair contribute through their association with inflammation and localized fluid retention. When tissue is stressed, repair processes involve increased blood flow, signaling activity, and fluid accumulation in the affected areas. This can raise measured weight temporarily. The increase does not indicate a change in stored energy. It reflects the system's response to tissue stress and its effort to restore structural integrity.

Inflammation more broadly can influence fluid balance and mass. Systemic or localized inflammatory responses can alter how fluid is retained, leading to short-term increases in weight. These responses may arise from physical stress, illness, or other internal conditions. They represent active system behavior, not failure or dysfunction, but they can obscure the interpretation of the scale when viewed in isolation.

Sleep disruption and stress signaling further affect short-term regulation. Changes in sleep quality and stress load can alter hormonal signaling patterns that influence fluid retention, appetite rhythm, and substrate allocation. These changes may not produce immediate shifts in stored energy, but they can modify fluid balance and digestive behavior in ways that are visible on the scale. The number moves, but the movement reflects regulatory adjustment rather than a clear directional change in storage.

Recovery state integrates many of these factors. When recovery is compromised, signaling patterns shift, resource allocation changes, and fluid regulation can become more variable. When recovery is stable, the system may still produce fluctuations as it continues to adjust to ongoing conditions. The presence of variability does not distinguish between these states on its own. It simply reflects that the system is active.

These sources of fluctuation do not operate in isolation. They often occur simultaneously, and their effects can overlap or offset each other. A reduction in glycogen and associated water may lower measured weight while an increase in inflammation-related fluid retention raises it. Digestive contents may increase mass at the same time that hydration shifts reduce it. The scale reports the net result of these overlapping processes. It does not display their individual contributions or their opposing directions.

This overlap is central to understanding variability. The number on the scale is the outcome of multiple processes moving at once, some increasing mass and others decreasing it. Because these processes operate on different timescales, the visible output can appear irregular when observed over short intervals. The irregularity is not random. It reflects the interaction of multiple regulated components.

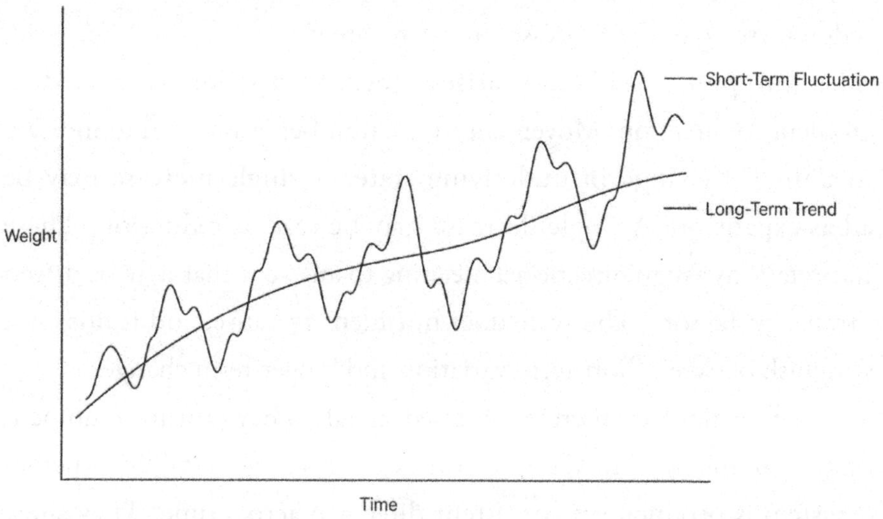

[Figure 4: Short-Term Fluctuation vs Long-Term Trend]

The contrast between fluctuation and trend becomes visible when readings are observed across time. Short-term measurements move up and down as these processes interact. Over longer intervals, a broader pattern begins to emerge as repeated conditions produce accumulated effects. The daily variability does not disappear, but it becomes contextualized within a larger trajectory.

Variability, in this sense, is not evidence of system failure. It is evidence of system activity. A responsive biological system must adjust continuously to maintain internal stability under changing conditions. It redistributes fluid, stores and releases energy, processes intake, repairs tissue, and adapts to stress. These actions create movement in the measured output because the output captures their combined effect.

A system that produced no variation at all would not necessarily be more stable; it might simply be less responsive to changing conditions. Stability does not require a flat output. It requires coordinated internal behavior that maintains functional integrity. That coordination often involves movement. The visible number reflects that movement because it is downstream of the processes that generate it.

The interpretive difficulty arises when fluctuation is treated as equivalent to direction. Movement in the number is assumed to indicate a meaningful change in underlying state. A single increase may be read as expansion. A single decrease may be read as reduction. These interpretations assign directional meaning to an event that may be driven by transient factors. The scale does not identify cause, and it does not distinguish between short-term variation and longer-term change.

Isolated readings are therefore limited signals. They capture a moment within a variable system. Without context, they cannot establish whether the system is producing a consistent direction across time. They show that the number moved. They do not show why it moved or whether the movement is part of a broader pattern.

Event interpretation overreads the scale by assuming that each reading carries full explanatory power. It treats the number as though it directly reflects underlying storage without considering the other components that contribute to total mass. This leads to conclusions that are sensitive to short-term variation and vulnerable to misinterpretation.

Trend provides a different form of information. It reflects repeated outputs observed across time, allowing transient fluctuations to be placed within a broader context. Trend does not eliminate variability, but it reduces the influence of individual fluctuations by integrating multiple readings. When the system is observed across enough time, the accumulated effects of intake, expenditure, signaling, recovery, and adaptation begin to shape a directional pattern that is more stable than any single reading.

This stability does not arise because the system becomes less complex. It arises because repeated observations allow the signal to be interpreted through time rather than through isolated events. Short-term changes continue to occur, but they become less dominant when viewed against a longer sequence of readings. The pattern provides a structure within which fluctuation can be understood.

Interpreting weight through trend aligns the signal with the nature of the system that produces it. The system operates continuously, integrating inputs and producing outputs over time. A single reading cannot capture that continuity. A pattern can approximate it by reflecting how the output behaves across multiple intervals.

The scale becomes more useful when its variability is understood in this way. The number remains a valid measurement of total mass, but its meaning is not assigned at the level of individual events. It is derived from patterns that emerge across time. Movement is acknowledged without being overinterpreted. Direction is identified through accumulation rather than through reaction.

This distinction preserves the value of the signal while protecting it from misinterpretation. The scale is neither dismissed nor treated as definitive in isolation. It is recognized as a variable output produced by a system with multiple interacting components. Its readings are informative when placed within context and less informative when treated as standalone events.

The central distinction follows from this structure. Fluctuation and trend are not the same kind of information. Fluctuation shows that the number moved. Trend shows whether the system is producing a directional pattern across time.

Intake Mechanism

Energy enters the system through intake, and that entry point carries immediate importance. Without intake, there is no incoming substrate to be processed, stored, or used. This makes intake a central input within the regulation of body weight. At the same time, intake does not operate independently. It does not arrive into an empty or neutral structure. It enters a system already defined by prior conditions, ongoing demands, signaling patterns, and adaptive history. This dual reality—intake as necessary input and intake as context-dependent input—requires a more precise frame than either dismissal or simplification.

Two common reductions tend to appear at this point. One treats intake as irrelevant because weight is complex, distributed, and influenced by many variables. The other treats intake as the complete explanation because energy enters the body through food. Both positions collapse under closer inspection. Intake matters because it introduces energy into the system, but it cannot be interpreted in isolation because the system receiving that energy determines how it is handled. Intake is not a detached cause. It is an input stream interacting with a regulated structure.

The body does not receive energy as an abstract number. Intake arrives through physical forms that require processing. Food carries volume, density, and composition. It engages digestive pathways that unfold over time. The act of intake initiates a sequence: ingestion, mechanical breakdown, enzymatic digestion, absorption, and distribution. These processes occur within a physiological environment that shapes their speed, efficiency, and downstream effects. Timing, meal structure, and the interaction of nutrients influence how energy becomes available to the system. None of these features operate independently of the body that receives them.

This is why intake cannot be reduced to quantity alone. Quantity is one dimension of the input, but it does not describe how that input is processed. Energy may enter quickly or slowly, in concentrated or distributed forms, under conditions of rest or demand, within states of high or low readiness for utilization. The same nominal amount can arrive under very different circumstances. The system does not respond only to how much energy enters. It responds to how that energy enters and to the context in which it arrives.

Before intake even reaches the point of processing, it is shaped by signals and constraints that determine when and how it occurs. Appetite and satiety function as regulatory signals within this process. They reflect internal conditions related to energy availability, hormonal signaling, and prior intake. Appetite is not a simple instruction. It is an expression of system state, influenced by recent intake, energy demand, sleep quality, stress load, and recovery condition. Satiety reflects the system's response to intake, contributing to the regulation of further consumption.

These signals do not operate in isolation from the broader environment. External constraints play a defining role in shaping intake patterns. Schedule, work demands, and social context influence when intake occurs. Food availability determines what forms of energy are accessible at a given time. Habit patterns develop through repeated exposure to specific conditions, creating structured tendencies that guide intake without requiring continuous decision-making. Environment organizes these elements, setting the boundaries within which intake takes place.

Stress and sleep further modify intake pressure by altering internal signaling. Elevated stress load can influence appetite through changes in hormonal regulation and perceived energy demand. Sleep disruption can affect hunger signals, satiety response, and overall regulatory balance. Fatigue alters decision-making capacity and the way environmental cues are processed. Recovery state integrates these influences, shaping both the internal signals that guide intake and the system's readiness to process incoming energy.

These forces demonstrate that intake is not simply chosen in isolation. It emerges from the interaction between internal signals and external constraints. The system produces pressure toward intake under certain conditions and reduces that pressure under others. Availability and structure then determine how that pressure is expressed. This interaction does not reduce intake to a fixed rule or a simple behavior. It positions intake as a dynamic input stream shaped by multiple influences before it even enters the body.

Once energy has entered the system, its meaning is determined by the state of the system receiving it. This receiving state is not static. It reflects prior intake patterns, current energy demand, glycogen status, activity level, sleep condition, stress load, and adaptive responses accumulated over time. Intake does not impose a fixed outcome. It is interpreted by the system through these existing conditions.

Glycogen status provides a clear example of this interaction. When glycogen stores are reduced, incoming energy may be directed toward replenishment. When glycogen stores are already elevated, the same intake may be handled differently, with less immediate allocation toward storage in that compartment. This does not require conscious direction. It is a function of system state guiding resource allocation.

Energy demand also influences how intake is processed. Periods of higher demand create conditions in which incoming energy is more likely to be used for immediate needs. Periods of lower demand alter that distribution. The system does not treat all intake identically because demand is not constant. It adjusts allocation based on current requirements and available resources.

Recovery state modifies this process further. When the system is in a state of repair or adaptation, incoming energy may be directed toward restoration processes. When recovery is constrained, signaling patterns may shift in ways that alter how energy is distributed. Stress load interacts with these dynamics, influencing hormonal signaling and resource prioritization. The same intake can therefore produce different downstream effects depending on whether the system is operating under stable, stressed, or recovery-focused conditions.

Insulin signaling and broader hormonal coordination play a central role in determining how intake is handled. These signals influence whether energy is directed toward immediate use, storage, or redistribution. They also interact with prior conditions, including recent intake and activity patterns. The system's sensitivity to these signals is not fixed. It adapts over time, meaning that identical inputs can be processed differently across different phases of system behavior.

Adaptation itself introduces another layer of complexity. Repeated patterns of intake and expenditure lead to adjustments in efficiency, signaling, and substrate use. These adjustments alter how future intake is processed. The system is not simply responding to the current input. It is responding as a system that has already adapted to prior inputs. This creates continuity across time, linking present intake to past conditions.

This continuity is why intake cannot be interpreted as a single event with a complete explanation. Each instance of intake is part of an ongoing sequence. It interacts with what came before and influences what follows. The system integrates these interactions over time, producing outputs that reflect accumulated behavior rather than isolated inputs. Weight, as a downstream output, emerges from this integration.

Because intake enters a system with these properties, it cannot be treated as a moral event. Moral framing treats the act of intake as though it carries inherent meaning independent of context. This approach detaches intake from the system that processes it and reduces it to a binary evaluation. Such evaluation does not align with the structure of the system. Intake is neither inherently corrective nor inherently disruptive. Its effect depends on how it is received, processed, and integrated within the broader regulatory environment.

Removing moral framing does not reduce the importance of intake. It clarifies its role. Intake matters because it introduces energy into the system, influencing storage, use, signaling, and subsequent regulation. At the same time, its meaning cannot be determined without reference to the system state in which it occurs. Treating intake as a moral category obscures this dependency and encourages interpretations that are disconnected from system behavior.

Intake also cannot be elevated to a complete explanation for weight. While it is a primary entry point for energy, it interacts with other processes that determine how that energy contributes to overall system behavior. Expenditure, storage, release, hormonal signaling, appetite regulation, recovery state, and adaptation all participate in shaping the outcome. Weight emerges from the interaction of these processes across time. Intake is one input among many, and its effect is mediated by the system as a whole.

This perspective maintains precision without oversimplification. It acknowledges that energy must enter the system for storage to occur, but it also recognizes that the path from intake to storage is not direct or uniform. The system can allocate incoming energy toward immediate use, storage in different forms, or redistribution across compartments. It can adjust efficiency, alter signaling patterns, and change its response based on prior conditions. These dynamics prevent intake from serving as a standalone explanation.

Understanding intake as an input stream rather than a fixed event allows it to be interpreted within this structure. The focus shifts from evaluating individual instances to examining how intake interacts with system state over time. Patterns of intake, shaped by signals and constraints, become more relevant than isolated occurrences. The system's response to those patterns, influenced by its current condition and adaptive history, determines how energy is integrated.

This approach also aligns intake with the temporal structure established in earlier mechanisms. Output is delayed because the system processes inputs over time. Variability arises because multiple processes contribute to the output simultaneously. Intake participates in both of these dynamics. It enters the system at specific moments, but its effects are distributed across time through processing, allocation, and adaptation. The visible output reflects this distribution rather than any single instance of intake.

The role of intake becomes clearer when it is placed within this framework. It is not irrelevant, and it is not complete. It is a necessary input that interacts with a regulated system. Its meaning is derived from that interaction. Without intake, there is no incoming energy to be processed. With intake, there is an input that must be interpreted by the system receiving it.

This leads to the governing distinction. Intake is an input, not a moral event. It matters because it enters the system. It becomes interpretable only when placed inside the system that receives and processes it.

Expenditure Mechanism

Energy leaves the system through use, but that use does not occur through a single pathway. It is not confined to moments of visible activity, nor does it operate as a clean subtraction that can be isolated from the rest of the system. Expenditure is often reduced to what can be seen—structured movement, deliberate exercise, or periods of physical effort. This narrowing is understandable because these forms of energy use are observable and discrete. They have a beginning and an end. They can be labeled as activity.

The body does not organize its energy use in that way. Energy is used continuously, whether activity is visible or not. The system maintains function across all states, including rest, movement, digestion, recovery, and adaptation. These processes operate simultaneously, each drawing from available energy to sustain internal stability. The visible portions of expenditure represent only one segment of a broader, distributed system.

Expenditure, in this sense, is not a single value. It is a composite of processes that operate at different intensities and across different timescales. Some are constant, providing the baseline conditions required for life. Others fluctuate in response to behavior, environment, and internal state. Together, they form the total energy use of the system. Understanding expenditure requires attention to this distribution rather than to any one component in isolation.

Resting function accounts for a substantial portion of this distribution. Even in the absence of deliberate movement, the body is not inactive.

Organ systems continue to operate without interruption. The heart maintains circulation, the lungs sustain respiration, and the nervous system coordinates signaling across tissues. Cellular processes continue to repair, replace, and maintain structural integrity. Temperature is regulated within a narrow range despite changes in the external environment. These processes require energy at all times.

This baseline use is often described as resting metabolism, but the term can obscure its complexity. It is not a passive state. It is continuous operation. The system does not suspend its functions between periods of activity. It sustains them, drawing on energy to preserve coherence and stability. The energy required for these processes does not appear as movement, but it is essential to the system's integrity. Without it, no other form of activity would be possible.

Beyond resting function, movement expands the range of energy use. Movement includes structured activity, but it is not limited to it. The body moves in ways that are not always consciously directed. Posture shifts, transitions between positions, walking through daily environments, and small adjustments in balance all require energy. These movements occur throughout the day, often without deliberate attention. They are part of the system's interaction with its environment.

This broader category of movement also includes spontaneous activity that varies with internal and external conditions. When energy availability is higher, movement may increase in ways that are not planned. When fatigue or stress is present, movement may decrease. Schedule, occupation, and environment shape how much movement occurs and in what form. These variations are not random. They reflect the system's response to current conditions and constraints.

Formal activity is one expression within this range. It is identifiable because it is structured and often intentional. However, it does not define the entirety of movement-related expenditure. The body continues to use energy outside these defined periods. Treating formal activity as the primary or only meaningful form of expenditure obscures the broader context in which energy is used.

Digestion introduces another layer of energy use. Processing intake requires work. Food must be broken down mechanically and chemically, nutrients must be absorbed, and metabolic pathways must handle incoming substrates. This process consumes energy as part of the system's effort to integrate new input. The energy cost of digestion varies with the characteristics of the intake, but its presence is consistent. Intake does not enter the system without being processed, and that processing contributes to overall expenditure.

Thermoregulation adds further demand. The body maintains internal temperature within a narrow range despite fluctuations in the external environment. This regulation requires energy. Heat must be produced or dissipated to preserve internal conditions. Changes in ambient temperature, clothing, activity level, and physiological state all influence the energy required to maintain thermal balance. These adjustments occur continuously, often without awareness, but they contribute to total energy use.

Recovery and repair extend the distribution of expenditure into periods that may appear inactive. When tissues are stressed or damaged, the system allocates resources to restoration. This includes protein synthesis, cellular repair, and the resolution of inflammation. These processes require energy. They may occur during rest or sleep, but they are active components of system maintenance. The energy directed toward recovery is part of the broader expenditure landscape.

These processes—resting function, movement, digestion, thermoregulation, and recovery—do not operate independently. They interact and overlap. Energy allocated to one process may influence what is available for another. The system continuously balances these demands, distributing resources in a way that maintains overall stability. Total energy use reflects this balancing process, not a single isolated action.

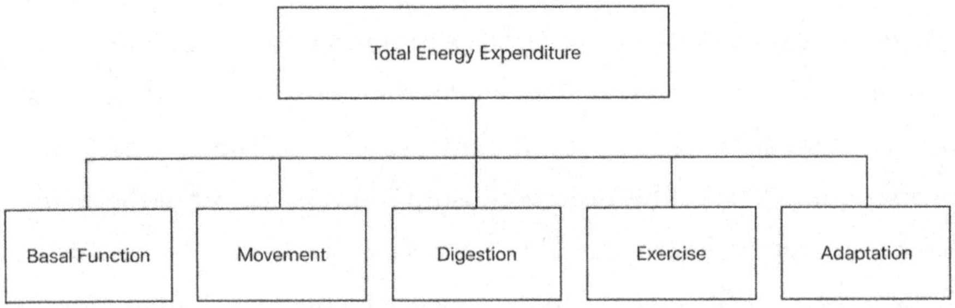

[Figure 5: Components of Expenditure]

The figure represents expenditure as a set of contributing processes rather than a single value. Resting function, movement, digestion, thermoregulation, and recovery each draw from the system's available energy. Their combined activity produces total expenditure. The proportions may shift, but the structure remains distributed.

This distribution also explains why expenditure is not fixed. The system does not operate at a constant level of energy use regardless of conditions. It adjusts in response to changes in intake, activity, body size, sleep, stress, and recovery state. These adjustments occur through multiple pathways, altering how energy is allocated and how efficiently processes operate.

When intake changes, the system may respond by modifying energy use. This does not imply a violation of energy balance. It reflects a shift within it. The system can alter spontaneous movement, adjust thermoregulatory demands, and modify efficiency in certain processes. These changes influence total expenditure without requiring a single, uniform adjustment across all components.

Activity level also influences expenditure, but not only through the direct cost of movement. Changes in activity can affect recovery demands, alter spontaneous movement patterns, and interact with signaling pathways that regulate energy use. The system integrates these changes, adjusting how energy is distributed across processes.

Body size contributes to baseline energy requirements. Larger systems require more energy to maintain function, while smaller systems require less. This relationship influences resting expenditure, but it also interacts with other variables. Changes in body composition and structure can alter how energy is used and allocated across processes.

Sleep and stress further shape expenditure by influencing signaling and resource allocation. Sleep disruption can affect recovery processes, hormonal regulation, and spontaneous movement. Stress can alter thermoregulation, fluid balance, and energy distribution. These influences do not operate in isolation. They interact with other components of the system, contributing to shifts in total energy use.

Adaptation provides a mechanism through which these adjustments persist over time. Repeated conditions—whether related to intake, activity, or environment—lead to changes in efficiency and allocation. The system becomes calibrated to its operating conditions. This calibration influences how future energy is used, altering the relationship between inputs and outputs.

Adaptive changes do not represent dysfunction. They are part of the system's effort to maintain stability under changing conditions. Efficiency may increase in some processes and decrease in others. Movement patterns may shift. Thermoregulatory demands may adjust. These changes affect total expenditure, but they do so within the framework of a responsive system.

Because expenditure is distributed and adaptive, it cannot be reduced to a single, stable number that remains constant across conditions. It varies with the state of the system and the demands placed upon it. This variability does not make expenditure unpredictable. It reflects structured responses to changes in input, environment, and internal state.

The interaction between intake and expenditure must be understood within this dynamic framework. Intake introduces energy into the system, and expenditure represents how that energy is used. Neither operates as a fixed quantity. Both are shaped by the same underlying processes of regulation, signaling, and adaptation. Energy balance, therefore, is not a simple exchange between two static values. It is the result of interacting variables that change over time.

Weight, as a downstream output, reflects the integration of these variables. It does not respond directly to isolated changes in intake or expenditure. It reflects how the system has processed those changes across time, incorporating storage, release, signaling, and adaptation. The variability and lag observed in weight are consistent with the distributed and dynamic nature of energy use.

Expenditure becomes more interpretable when it is understood as a process rather than a fixed value. The body uses energy continuously, across multiple domains, and adjusts that use in response to changing conditions. Visible activity is one part of this process, but it does not define it. The system's energy use extends beyond what can be observed directly.

The central distinction follows from this structure. Energy expenditure is dynamic, not fixed. It is the system's distributed use of energy across resting function, movement, digestion, thermoregulation, recovery, and adaptation.

Storage Mechanism

Storage is often misread because it becomes visible through body mass. Once stored energy contributes to weight, it can be treated as though it were a problem separate from the system that produced it. The visible result is isolated from the function that made it necessary. In that narrowed view, storage appears as excess, accumulation, or failure. The system-level view begins elsewhere. Storage exists because energy arrival and energy demand are not synchronized moment by moment.

Intake occurs in episodes. Energy use continues across time. The body must sustain organ function, cellular work, circulation, respiration, nervous system activity, temperature regulation, movement, digestion, immune activity, recovery, and repair even when no new energy is entering. Demand does not pause between intake events. It rises and falls, but it does not disappear. A system that could only use energy at the moment it arrived would be structurally fragile. It would depend on continuous intake to support continuous function.

Storage resolves that mismatch. It allows energy to be held when availability exceeds immediate demand and accessed later when demand exceeds incoming supply. This makes storage part of temporal regulation. It connects periods of energy arrival with periods of energy use. It gives the system continuity across gaps, variation, and changing conditions. Storage is not an exception to normal function. It is one of the ways normal function remains continuous.

Energy buffering is the central role of storage. Buffering does not mean inactivity. It means the system can absorb variation without losing stability. Intake may arrive in a concentrated period, while expenditure continues across hours. Activity may rise after intake or long after it. Recovery may require resources during sleep. Thermoregulation may demand energy in response to environmental change. Repair may become more active after tissue stress. Storage allows energy to be distributed across these shifting demands instead of being tied only to the timing of intake.

Incoming energy can move through several routes. Some may be directed toward immediate use, supporting current cellular work, organ function, movement, digestion, or temperature regulation. Some may be stored as glycogen, a limited and relatively accessible form of short-term energy buffering. Some may be stored as fat, a more energy-dense form suited to longer-term buffering. Some may support repair and recovery demands. Some may be held for later release when availability, demand, and signaling conditions change.

These routes are not mutually exclusive. The system does not choose one pathway in isolation while shutting down all others. Energy allocation is distributed. Immediate use, storage, repair, and later release can overlap within the same broader state. Routing depends on current demand, prior intake, glycogen status, hormonal signaling, activity, sleep, stress load, recovery state, and adaptive history. The body is not passively filled by incoming energy. It actively allocates substrate in relation to conditions already present.

Glycogen serves a short-term buffering role. It is limited compared with longer-term storage, but it is useful because it is relatively accessible and closely connected to short-term fuel availability. Liver glycogen helps support blood glucose regulation between intake events. Muscle glycogen supports local muscular demand. These stores can shift more quickly than longer-term storage compartments because they are tied to recent intake, recent demand, and current availability.

Glycogen also carries a visible relationship to water. Stored glycogen is associated with retained water, so changes in glycogen status can move scale weight quickly. When glycogen is reduced, associated water may decrease. When glycogen is replenished, associated water may increase. This is one reason short-term weight movement can occur without a corresponding change in longer-term stored energy. The scale registers the mass change, but it does not identify whether the movement reflects glycogen, water, fat storage, digestion, inflammation, or another contributor.

Fat storage serves a different system role. It is larger in capacity and more energy-dense, making it suited to longer-term buffering. It allows energy to be held across extended intervals and accessed when availability or demand changes. This role is real and should not be minimized. At the same time, it should not be moralized. Fat storage is not a moral category. It is one form of energy buffering within a system that must manage availability across time.

The distinction between glycogen and fat storage matters because they behave differently. Glycogen is more limited, more closely tied to short-term availability, and more visibly linked to water shifts. Fat storage is more energy-dense and slower to change in a way that is clearly visible through weight. Both belong to energy regulation. Neither explains the entire system alone.

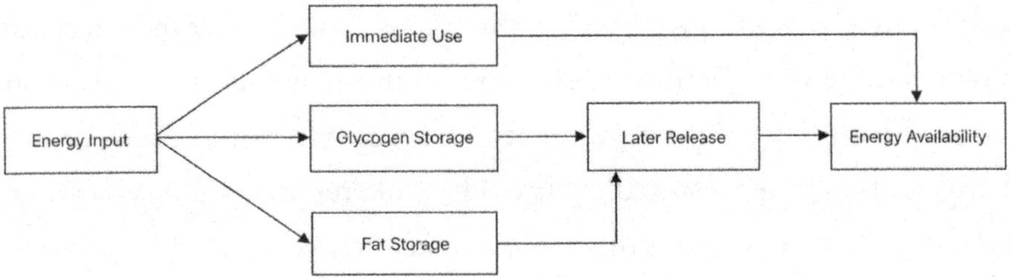

[Figure 6: Energy Storage and Release]

The figure represents energy input moving toward immediate use, glycogen storage, fat storage, repair and recovery demands, and later release. These routes are not separate judgments about the input. They are coordinated pathways through which the system manages demand, availability, buffering, and continuity.

Storage is meaningful because release is possible. Stored energy would have little functional value if it could never be accessed. Release is not the moral opposite of storage. It is the paired function that makes storage useful. The system stores when conditions support holding energy and releases when conditions support access. Both actions belong to the same mechanism.

This pairing is coordinated by demand and signaling. When immediate energy demand rises, stored substrate may become more relevant. When incoming energy is available, the system may reduce reliance on stored sources and allocate new substrate toward use, storage, or repair. When intake is absent, release can support continued function. When recovery demands are high, allocation may shift toward restoration. Storage and release are not separate states with fixed meanings. They are movements within a regulated system.

Hormonal signaling helps coordinate these movements. Insulin participates in directing incoming energy toward use and storage when substrate is available. Other signals influence mobilization, appetite, stress response, sleep-related regulation, and recovery allocation. These signals do not act as isolated switches. They operate as part of a coordinated network that interprets availability, demand, and prior conditions. No single hormone explains storage dynamics by itself. The relevant feature is coordination.

Prior conditions shape that coordination. The system does not respond to today's intake as if yesterday did not happen. Existing glycogen status, recent activity, sleep quality, stress load, recovery state, and adaptive history all influence routing. If glycogen stores are lower, incoming substrate may be handled differently than when glycogen stores are already higher. If activity demand has been elevated, allocation may shift toward replenishment and repair. If recovery is constrained, signaling and fluid regulation may alter how storage dynamics appear externally.

Recovery and repair require resources. Tissue maintenance, immune activity, and cellular restoration all draw from available energy. Some incoming energy may support these processes directly. Stored energy may also contribute when conditions require access to internal reserves. This means storage cannot be interpreted only through the lens of visible mass. It also supports maintenance processes that may not show up as immediate change on the scale.

Stress and sleep influence storage dynamics by altering the signaling environment in which allocation occurs. Stress load can affect fluid regulation, appetite signaling, substrate handling, and recovery prioritization. Sleep disruption can influence hormonal rhythm, recovery quality, and short-term regulation. These influences may alter storage and release indirectly, not by creating one simple outcome, but by changing the conditions under which energy is allocated.

Adaptation extends this process across time. Repeated patterns of intake, expenditure, stress, sleep, and recovery can change how the system handles future inputs. Efficiency may shift. Spontaneous movement may change. Recovery demands may accumulate or resolve. Substrate use may recalibrate. These adaptations do not erase energy balance; they change the variables operating inside it. Storage dynamics are therefore historical as well as immediate. They reflect present conditions shaped by prior conditions.

Weight reflects storage dynamics, but imperfectly. A change in scale weight may involve storage, but it may also involve glycogen-linked water, digestive contents, fluid shifts, inflammation, recovery-related retention, changes in substrate availability, or delayed release and storage effects. The scale compresses all of these into one visible output. It does not identify the compartment or pathway responsible for the movement.

This is why short-term increases should not be automatically interpreted as fat storage, and short-term decreases should not be automatically interpreted as fat reduction or stored energy release. A rapid increase may reflect water associated with glycogen, digestive contents, inflammation, or recovery-related fluid retention. A rapid decrease may reflect fluid release, glycogen reduction, or gastrointestinal change. These movements are real, but their meaning is limited without context.

Longer-term storage changes can influence weight, but they usually appear through the same delayed and variable output described earlier. Storage is processed internally before it becomes visible externally. The output arrives after lag, mixed with other contributors. Weight may eventually reflect changes in storage pattern, but it does not report storage activity cleanly in real time.

This does not make weight useless. It means the signal must be interpreted according to what it can and cannot show. Weight can indicate that total mass has changed. It cannot, by itself, separate glycogen from water, fat storage from fluid retention, digestion from recovery, or short-term fluctuation from longer-term direction. Storage affects weight, but weight is not a direct window into storage.

Storage belongs inside system interpretation, not moral interpretation. It is part of how the body manages mismatch between energy arrival and energy demand. It supports continuity when intake is absent, buffers availability when immediate need is lower, and allows later access when conditions change. Its meaning depends on routing, signaling, demand, recovery, stress, sleep, activity, and adaptation.

The central correction is structural. Storage is a system function, not an isolated problem. It allows energy to be buffered, held, accessed, and released across time.

Hormonal Coordination Mechanism

Storage is often misread because it becomes visible through body mass. Once stored energy contributes to weight, it can be treated as though it were a problem separate from the system that produced it. The visible result is isolated from the function that made it necessary. In that narrowed view, storage appears as excess, accumulation, or failure. The system-level view begins elsewhere. Storage exists because energy arrival and energy demand are not synchronized moment by moment.

Intake occurs in episodes. Energy use continues across time. The body must sustain organ function, cellular work, circulation, respiration, nervous system activity, temperature regulation, movement, digestion, immune activity, recovery, and repair even when no new energy is entering. Demand does not pause between intake events. It rises and falls, but it does not disappear. A system that could only use energy at the moment it arrived would be structurally fragile. It would depend on continuous intake to support continuous function.

Storage resolves that mismatch. It allows energy to be held when availability exceeds immediate demand and accessed later when demand exceeds incoming supply. This makes storage part of temporal regulation. It connects periods of energy arrival with periods of energy use. It gives the system continuity across gaps, variation, and changing conditions. Storage is not an exception to normal function. It is one of the ways normal function remains continuous.

Energy buffering is the central role of storage. Buffering does not mean inactivity. It means the system can absorb variation without losing stability. Intake may arrive in a concentrated period, while expenditure continues across hours. Activity may rise after intake or long after it. Recovery may require resources during sleep. Thermoregulation may demand energy in response to environmental change. Repair may become more active after tissue stress. Storage allows energy to be distributed across these shifting demands instead of being tied only to the timing of intake.

Incoming energy can move through several routes. Some may be directed toward immediate use, supporting current cellular work, organ function, movement, digestion, or temperature regulation. Some may be stored as glycogen, a limited and relatively accessible form of short-term energy buffering. Some may be stored as fat, a more energy-dense form suited to longer-term buffering. Some may support repair and recovery demands. Some may be held for later release when availability, demand, and signaling conditions change.

These routes are not mutually exclusive. The system does not choose one pathway in isolation while shutting down all others. Energy allocation is distributed. Immediate use, storage, repair, and later release can overlap within the same broader state. Routing depends on current demand, prior intake, glycogen status, hormonal signaling, activity, sleep, stress load, recovery state, and adaptive history. The body is not passively filled by incoming energy. It actively allocates substrate in relation to conditions already present.

Glycogen serves a short-term buffering role. It is limited compared with longer-term storage, but it is useful because it is relatively accessible and closely connected to short-term fuel availability. Liver glycogen helps support blood glucose regulation between intake events. Muscle glycogen supports local muscular demand. These stores can shift more quickly than longer-term storage compartments because they are tied to recent intake, recent demand, and current availability.

Glycogen also carries a visible relationship to water. Stored glycogen is associated with retained water, so changes in glycogen status can move scale weight quickly. When glycogen is reduced, associated water may decrease. When glycogen is replenished, associated water may increase. This is one reason short-term weight movement can occur without a corresponding change in longer-term stored energy. The scale registers the mass change, but it does not identify whether the movement reflects glycogen, water, fat storage, digestion, inflammation, or another contributor.

Fat storage serves a different system role. It is larger in capacity and more energy-dense, making it suited to longer-term buffering. It allows energy to be held across extended intervals and accessed when availability or demand changes. This role is real and should not be minimized. At the same time, it should not be moralized. Fat storage is not a moral category. It is one form of energy buffering within a system that must manage availability across time.

The distinction between glycogen and fat storage matters because they behave differently. Glycogen is more limited, more closely tied to short-term availability, and more visibly linked to water shifts. Fat storage is more energy-dense and slower to change in a way that is clearly visible through weight. Both belong to energy regulation. Neither explains the entire system alone.

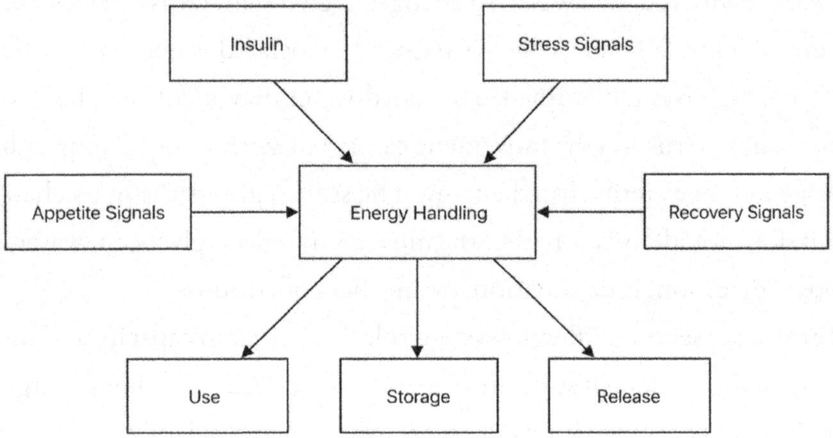

[Figure 7 — Hormonal Coordination]

The figure represents energy input moving toward immediate use, glycogen storage, fat storage, repair and recovery demands, and later release. These routes are not separate judgments about the input. They are coordinated pathways through which the system manages demand, availability, buffering, and continuity.

Storage is meaningful because release is possible. Stored energy would have little functional value if it could never be accessed. Release is not the moral opposite of storage. It is the paired function that makes storage useful. The system stores when conditions support holding energy and releases when conditions support access. Both actions belong to the same mechanism.

This pairing is coordinated by demand and signaling. When immediate energy demand rises, stored substrate may become more relevant. When incoming energy is available, the system may reduce reliance on stored sources and allocate new substrate toward use, storage, or repair. When intake is absent, release can support continued function. When recovery demands are high, allocation may shift toward restoration. Storage and release are not separate states with fixed meanings. They are movements within a regulated system.

Hormonal signaling helps coordinate these movements. Insulin participates in directing incoming energy toward use and storage when substrate is available. Other signals influence mobilization, appetite, stress response, sleep-related regulation, and recovery allocation. These signals do not act as isolated switches. They operate as part of a coordinated network that interprets availability, demand, and prior conditions. No single hormone explains storage dynamics by itself. The relevant feature is coordination.

Prior conditions shape that coordination. The system does not respond to today's intake as if yesterday did not happen. Existing glycogen status, recent activity, sleep quality, stress load, recovery state, and adaptive history all influence routing. If glycogen stores are lower, incoming substrate may be handled differently than when glycogen stores are already higher. If activity demand has been elevated, allocation may shift toward replenishment and repair. If recovery is constrained, signaling and fluid regulation may alter how storage dynamics appear externally.

Recovery and repair require resources. Tissue maintenance, immune activity, and cellular restoration all draw from available energy. Some incoming energy may support these processes directly. Stored energy may also contribute when conditions require access to internal reserves. This means storage cannot be interpreted only through the lens of visible mass. It also supports maintenance processes that may not show up as immediate change on the scale.

Stress and sleep influence storage dynamics by altering the signaling environment in which allocation occurs. Stress load can affect fluid regulation, appetite signaling, substrate handling, and recovery prioritization. Sleep disruption can influence hormonal rhythm, recovery quality, and short-term regulation. These influences may alter storage and release indirectly, not by creating one simple outcome, but by changing the conditions under which energy is allocated.

Adaptation extends this process across time. Repeated patterns of intake, expenditure, stress, sleep, and recovery can change how the system handles future inputs. Efficiency may shift. Spontaneous movement may change. Recovery demands may accumulate or resolve. Substrate use may recalibrate. These adaptations do not erase energy balance; they change the variables operating inside it. Storage dynamics are therefore historical as well as immediate. They reflect present conditions shaped by prior conditions.

Weight reflects storage dynamics, but imperfectly. A change in scale weight may involve storage, but it may also involve glycogen-linked water, digestive contents, fluid shifts, inflammation, recovery-related retention, changes in substrate availability, or delayed release and storage effects. The scale compresses all of these into one visible output. It does not identify the compartment or pathway responsible for the movement.

This is why short-term increases should not be automatically interpreted as fat storage, and short-term decreases should not be automatically interpreted as fat reduction or stored energy release. A rapid increase may reflect water associated with glycogen, digestive contents, inflammation, or recovery-related fluid retention. A rapid decrease may reflect fluid release, glycogen reduction, or gastrointestinal change. These movements are real, but their meaning is limited without context.

Longer-term storage changes can influence weight, but they usually appear through the same delayed and variable output described earlier. Storage is processed internally before it becomes visible externally. The output arrives after lag, mixed with other contributors. Weight may eventually reflect changes in storage pattern, but it does not report storage activity cleanly in real time.

This does not make weight useless. It means the signal must be interpreted according to what it can and cannot show. Weight can indicate that total mass has changed. It cannot, by itself, separate glycogen from water, fat storage from fluid retention, digestion from recovery, or short-term fluctuation from longer-term direction. Storage affects weight, but weight is not a direct window into storage.

Storage belongs inside system interpretation, not moral interpretation. It is part of how the body manages mismatch between energy arrival and energy demand. It supports continuity when intake is absent, buffers availability when immediate need is lower, and allows later access when conditions change. Its meaning depends on routing, signaling, demand, recovery, stress, sleep, activity, and adaptation.

The central correction is structural. Storage is a system function, not an isolated problem. It allows energy to be buffered, held, accessed, and released across time.

Appetite Regulation Mechanism

Appetite is often interpreted morally before it is understood structurally. Hunger is treated as something to defeat. Satiety is treated as proof of control. Cravings are treated as weakness. Intake pressure is treated as lack of discipline. In this frame, appetite becomes evidence about character rather than information about system state.

That interpretation removes appetite from the conditions that produce it. It treats hunger, satiety, and cravings as isolated personal events, when they are better understood as signals emerging from regulation. Appetite is not a single feeling and not a simple behavioral flaw. It is a signal environment shaped by energy availability, prior intake, sleep, stress, recovery demand, metabolic state, routine, reward exposure, and environmental cues. It belongs inside the same system that regulates intake, expenditure, storage, release, and adaptation.

Appetite is not a character test. It is part of regulation. Its function is not to provide moral evidence about the person experiencing it. Its function is to help organize intake pressure around perceived need, availability, timing, memory, and constraint. Sometimes those signals are clear. Sometimes they are noisy. Sometimes hunger, satiety, cravings, and environmental cues align. At other times, they move in different directions because they arise from different parts of the regulatory environment.

Hunger is the most familiar part of appetite, but it is not simply stomach emptiness. Mechanical emptiness can contribute, but hunger is shaped by a broader set of signals. Nutrient availability, glucose availability, hormonal signaling, prior intake, recent expenditure, sleep state, stress load, recovery demand, learned meal timing, and environmental exposure can all influence hunger. The system does not merely wait until the stomach is empty and then produce a signal. It interprets availability, demand, and pattern.

This anticipatory quality matters. Appetite can rise in expectation of intake because the system has learned timing. Repeated patterns create regulatory expectations. If intake has often occurred at a certain time or in a certain context, hunger may appear before a measurable energy need becomes obvious. This is not irrationality. It is pattern-based regulation. The system prepares for expected intake because past conditions have shaped present signaling.

Hunger can also intensify when energy availability is reduced or when demand rises. Recent expenditure, inadequate recovery, or prior restriction can alter the pressure surrounding intake. The signal may become more persistent because the system is responding to perceived scarcity, increased demand, or disrupted rhythm. Hunger in this sense is not weakness. It is a signal of system state, shaped by the relationship between availability and demand.

Satiety is similarly more complex than fullness. Fullness is partly mechanical, reflecting volume and distension within the digestive tract. Satiety is regulatory. It depends on digestive signaling, nutrient sensing, absorption, hormonal response, glucose availability, prior energy state, sleep, stress, prior restriction, meal timing patterns, and metabolic context. A full stomach and a durable satiety signal are not identical conditions.

Satiety may be delayed when the system has not yet registered incoming energy fully. It may be shortened when prior restriction, sleep disruption, elevated stress, or high recovery demand alters the signal environment. It may feel unstable when nutrient availability, reward exposure, or routine cues continue to generate intake pressure despite physical fullness. These differences do not make satiety defective. They show that satiety is not a simple volume gauge. It is the system's interpretation of intake within context.

Glucose availability and nutrient sensing help inform this interpretation. When available substrate changes, appetite signals may shift. The system monitors incoming energy, circulating availability, storage access, and demand. These signals help shape hunger and satiety, but they do not explain appetite alone. Glucose availability interacts with insulin, stress signaling, sleep rhythm, expenditure demand, recovery state, and prior intake. No single signal fully explains hunger or satiety because appetite emerges from combined interpretation.

Sleep is one of the conditions that changes that interpretation. Sleep influences appetite rhythm, stress response, reward sensitivity, recovery quality, and hunger-satiety signaling. When sleep is disrupted, the signal environment changes. Hunger may become more pronounced, satiety may become less stable, reward cues may become more salient, and intake pressure may become harder to interpret. This is not a moral shift. It is a regulatory shift created by altered recovery and signaling conditions.

Stress also changes appetite by changing system state. Stress-related signaling can alter glucose availability, appetite pressure, fluid regulation, reward sensitivity, routine stability, and recovery allocation. Under stress, the system may prioritize readiness, availability, or short-term response. Appetite may intensify, become irregular, or shift toward cues and routines that have been repeatedly paired with relief, availability, or reward. Stress does not provide a single explanation for weight or appetite, but it modifies the conditions under which appetite signals are produced.

Cravings belong inside this same framework. A craving is directed intake pressure, not a moral failure. It may arise without obvious stomach hunger because appetite is not limited to digestive emptiness. Reward learning, repeated exposure, stress load, sleep disruption, prior restriction, energy pressure, routine, environmental cues, and associations between context and intake can all contribute. A craving indicates that a specific signal pattern has become active. It does not establish weakness, failure, or lack of control.

Reward and routine shape cravings through repetition. Certain times can become associated with intake. Certain places can increase cue exposure. Certain activities can become linked with eating through repeated pairing. Environmental cues can make specific intake patterns more salient before conscious decision-making begins. These cues do not override the entire system, but they participate in the signal environment. Appetite responds to context because context has become part of the pattern the system recognizes.

Prior restriction can intensify this pressure. When the system has experienced reduced availability, appetite signals may become stronger. Hunger may rise, cravings may become more salient, attention to food may increase, and satiety may be harder to sustain. This response reflects regulation under perceived constraint. The system carries history. Appetite does not reset cleanly at every moment as though prior intake patterns, energy pressure, and adaptive responses never occurred.

Recovery demand adds another layer. Repair, immune activity, cellular restoration, and recovery from exertion or stress require resources. When the system is under recovery load, appetite signals may shift because resource demand has changed. This does not mean appetite precisely identifies the exact recovery need. It means recovery participates in the broader regulation of intake pressure. Energy availability, tissue maintenance, and restoration are connected through signaling, even when the resulting appetite signal feels nonspecific.

Intake pressure is the convergence of these influences. It includes hunger, satiety, cravings, reward, routine, availability, sleep, stress, energy demand, prior restriction, recovery demand, and environment. It is not reducible to one sensation. It is the total pressure surrounding intake before intake occurs. Under stable conditions, that pressure may be relatively predictable. Under strain, it may become stronger, noisier, more persistent, more cue-sensitive, or harder to interpret.

This is regulation under load, not evidence of defect. When sleep is disrupted, stress is elevated, recovery demand is high, energy availability is low, routines are unstable, or cues are frequent, the appetite signal environment changes. Hunger and cravings may intensify while satiety may become less durable. Environmental cues may become more prominent. Repeated patterns may carry more influence. The system is still regulating, but it is regulating under constraint.

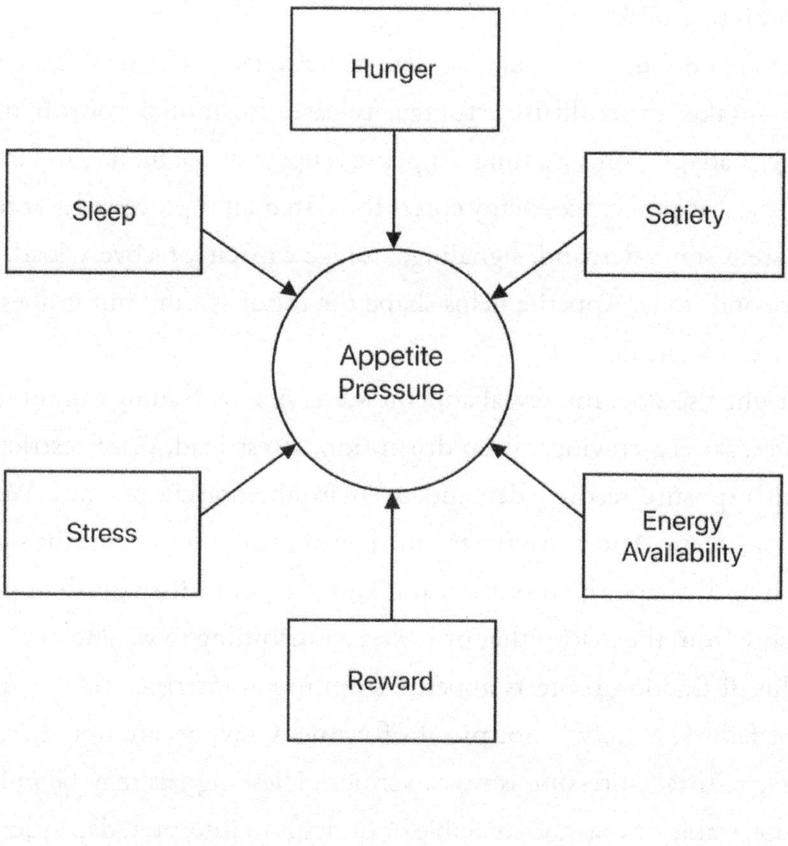

[Figure 8: Appetite Regulation]

The figure represents appetite pressure as a central node shaped by hunger, satiety, sleep, stress, energy availability, reward, routine, environmental cues, prior restriction, and recovery demand. These influences converge before intake occurs, forming the signal environment that shapes the input stream.

Appetite influences weight regulation because it shapes intake pressure. Intake is one of the major inputs into the weight regulation system, and appetite helps determine the conditions under which that input occurs. Hunger, satiety, cravings, reward, and routine can influence when intake becomes more likely, how persistent the pressure feels, and how the system responds to availability.

But appetite does not directly determine weight. Weight still emerges from intake, expenditure, storage, release, hormonal coordination, recovery, adaptation, and time. Appetite is upstream of intake, and intake is only one input. Once energy enters the system, it is processed according to system state, demand, signaling, storage capacity, recovery load, and prior conditions. Appetite helps shape the input stream, but it does not define the entire output.

Weight also does not reveal appetite state. A scale reading cannot show hunger, satiety, cravings, sleep disruption, stress load, prior restriction, reward exposure, recovery demand, or environmental cue pressure. Weight is downstream. Appetite is upstream. The output cannot name the signals that helped shape the input stream, and it cannot distinguish appetite pressure from the many other processes contributing to weight.

This distinction protects appetite from moral interpretation. Hunger is not failure. Satiety is not proof of virtue. Cravings are not character evidence. Intake pressure is not a verdict. These signals may be mild or intense, stable or noisy, predictable or difficult to interpret, depending on the conditions shaping them.

Appetite belongs inside system interpretation, not moral interpretation. It reflects regulation across energy availability, prior intake, sleep, stress, recovery demand, reward, routine, environment, metabolic state, and adaptation. Appetite is not a character test. It is part of regulation. Hunger, satiety, and cravings become interpretable only when placed inside the conditions that shape them.

Adaptation Mechanism

The body does not respond to each input as if it were isolated from history. Every meal, interval without intake, activity period, stress episode, sleep disruption, and recovery demand enters a system already shaped by what came before. The present state is not empty. It carries prior conditions forward through appetite pressure, expenditure patterns, substrate availability, storage and release dynamics, hormonal signaling, fluid regulation, recovery state, and adaptive calibration.

This continuity matters because weight regulation is not built from disconnected events. The system does not reset completely between days, meals, workouts, fasting intervals, or nights of sleep. It integrates repeated exposures into its operating state. What appears to be a current response is often the result of a current input meeting a history-shaped system. The input may be recent, but the receiving state is cumulative.

Adaptation is the process by which repeated conditions alter that receiving state. It is a form of calibration. When conditions repeat, the system adjusts appetite signals, energy availability, expenditure patterns, substrate handling, storage access, recovery allocation, and fluid regulation around those conditions. These adjustments may make weight response less immediate or less linear, but they are not automatically evidence of damage, dysfunction, or irrational resistance.

Adaptation is also not automatically beneficial. It is responsiveness. A system can adapt to conditions that support stability, and it can adapt to conditions that increase strain. The point is not to label adaptation as good or bad. The point is to recognize that repeated conditions change the operating context. Once the operating context changes, future inputs no longer enter the same system.

Repeated intake patterns are one way this occurs. Repeated low intake relative to demand may alter appetite pressure, perceived energy availability, expenditure patterns, storage access, recovery allocation, and spontaneous movement. Hunger signals may become more prominent. Energy use may shift in some domains. Recovery may compete more strongly for available resources. The system begins responding not only to the current intake event, but to the pattern of reduced availability it has repeatedly encountered.

Repeated higher intake can also alter response, but through a different pattern. Greater recurring availability may influence routing, storage dynamics, glycogen status, appetite rhythm, substrate handling, and perceived energy availability. The system may allocate incoming substrate differently depending on current demand, storage state, recovery load, and prior exposure. Higher intake is not a moral category. It is a condition the system processes and may adapt around when repeated.

Irregular intake adds another form of adaptation because timing itself becomes less predictable. When energy arrival varies substantially, hunger, satiety, and cravings may become less stable. The system has fewer consistent patterns around which to anticipate intake. Appetite timing can become noisier, and the interpretation of hunger or satiety can become less clear. This is not a character issue. It is a signal environment shaped by inconsistent availability.

Activity and movement patterns create their own adaptive context. Repeated inactivity can alter total expenditure, spontaneous movement, energy demand, substrate use, and the relationship between intake and storage. Lower movement demand changes the system's operating requirements. It may reduce some energy demands while changing how intake is routed through storage, use, and release. Inactivity should not be moralized; it is a repeated condition with physiological consequences inside the energy system.

Increased training or repeated physical demand produces a different set of adjustments. Repeated demand can raise recovery requirements, alter appetite pressure, increase repair needs, change substrate use, and create compensation pressure elsewhere in the system. The visible activity is only one component. The system must also manage tissue stress, restoration, fuel replenishment, sleep interaction, and the distribution of resources after the activity has ended.

This is why activity adaptation extends beyond the direct cost of movement. A period of physical demand may increase expenditure during the activity, but the total system response includes recovery allocation, appetite signaling, fluid shifts, glycogen dynamics, and possible changes in spontaneous movement. The body adapts not only to the movement itself, but to the recurring demand pattern surrounding that movement.

Fasting intervals can also become part of adaptation when they repeat as a timing structure. In this context, fasting means recurring input absence or a repeated pattern of intake timing, not a guaranteed outcome. The system may adapt around the rhythm of availability and absence by changing appetite timing, storage access, release patterns, perceived availability, and compensation pressure.

The same interval may be handled differently depending on prior state. A repeated interval occurring within stable sleep, sufficient recovery, low stress load, and consistent intake history is not the same signal as the same interval occurring under high stress, disrupted sleep, elevated recovery demand, or prior low availability. The timing may look identical from the outside, but the receiving state differs. Fasting intervals do not guarantee one output. They become part of the pattern the system interprets and adapts around.

Stress and sleep disruption alter adaptation by changing the signal environment. Repeated stress load can influence glucose availability, appetite pressure, fluid regulation, recovery allocation, expenditure patterns, and readiness signaling. Stress signals can shift the system toward immediate availability or resource prioritization. This does not make stress a moral failure or a single explanation for weight. It makes stress one repeated condition that can alter regulation over time.

Sleep disruption changes the system through recovery and signaling. Repeated disruption can alter appetite rhythm, stress response, glucose handling, fluid balance, recovery quality, and weight variability. The system may carry incomplete recovery forward, changing how it responds to intake, activity, and stress the next day. Over time, repeated sleep disruption can make the output more variable because the internal conditions producing that output are less stable.

Stress and sleep can also reinforce each other. Stress can interfere with recovery, and disrupted recovery can increase stress signaling. Together, they can change the context in which intake, expenditure, storage, and release occur. The system is still regulating, but it is regulating under altered conditions. Appetite may become noisier, fluid regulation may shift, recovery demands may accumulate, and expenditure patterns may change.

The central mechanism becomes clear when the same input appears under different prior states. The same meal after stable intake may be handled differently than the same meal after repeated low availability. The food itself may be identical, but appetite pressure, glycogen status, perceived availability, hormonal signaling, and storage-release dynamics may not be. The input is the same only on the surface.

The same activity can also produce different outputs depending on recovery state. Under strong recovery, the system may absorb the demand with less disruption. Under accumulated recovery strain, the same activity may increase repair demands, fluid retention, appetite pressure, or compensation elsewhere in expenditure. The movement may look identical, but the system receiving it is different.

The same fasting interval can also differ by context. Under lower stress and stable prior conditions, it may be one timing input within a broader pattern. Under high stress, disrupted sleep, or prior low availability, the same interval may interact with a more strained signal environment. The output may differ because the interval is not acting alone. It is being interpreted through current system state.

The same sleep disruption can likewise produce different consequences depending on history. One disrupted night after stable sleep may be buffered differently than the same disruption after repeated sleep loss. In the second case, recovery state, stress signaling, appetite rhythm, and fluid regulation may already be altered. The input is similar, but the accumulated context changes the response.

Current output is therefore partly historical. Weight reflects not only recent behavior, but the receiving state produced by repeated prior conditions. A scale reading may be delayed because internal processing takes time. It may fluctuate because multiple components contribute to total mass. Adaptation adds another layer: the system's response pattern itself can change over time.

This is why current weight response cannot be read as a direct verdict on the most recent event. A change may reflect accumulated intake patterns, altered expenditure, recovery strain, stress load, sleep disruption, glycogen status, fluid regulation, storage-release dynamics, or appetite pressure shaped over time. Recent behavior matters, but it enters a system that has already been calibrated by earlier conditions.

Weight stability is historical, not merely immediate. Long-term patterns emerge from repeated conditions and the adaptations they generate. Intake, expenditure, storage, release, appetite, hormonal coordination, activity, stress, sleep, recovery, and environment all participate across time. Stability is produced by accumulated system behavior, not by one isolated input.

Isolated events are weaker evidence because they do not reveal the state into which they entered. A single meal, day of movement, fasting interval, stressful episode, or disrupted night may matter, but its meaning becomes clearer only when placed inside the longer pattern. Repetition changes interpretation. Pattern reveals the operating context that a single event cannot show.

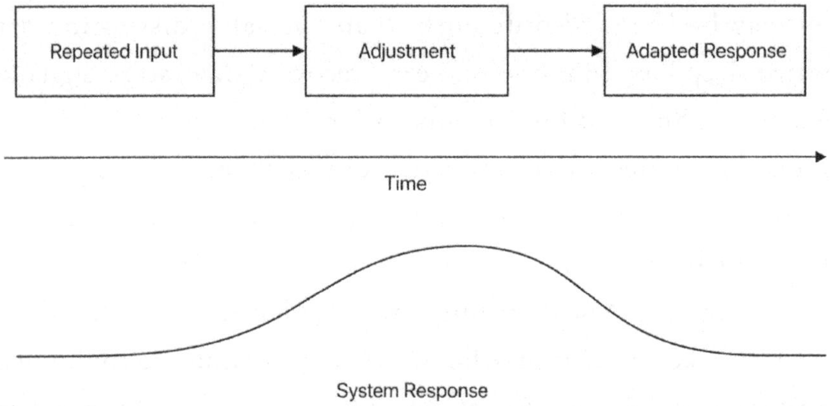

[Figure 9: Adaptation Over Time]

The figure represents repeated inputs leading to internal adjustment and then to an adapted response. The same input appears again, but it is no longer received by the same system state. Prior conditions have changed the receiving state, so the output may change as well.

Adaptation makes weight regulation historical rather than merely immediate. The system carries forward what it has repeatedly experienced through appetite pressure, expenditure patterns, storage and release dynamics, recovery allocation, signaling, substrate handling, and fluid regulation. The same input can produce different outputs after adaptation because the system receiving the input has changed.

Compensation Mechanism

Systems often respond to change by offsetting it. A change in one variable does not leave the rest of the system unchanged, because the body is not a static equation in which intake or activity changes while every other variable remains frozen. When intake changes, appetite may change. When activity changes, fatigue and recovery demand may change. When energy availability or demand shifts abruptly, spontaneous movement, fluid regulation, storage access, substrate handling, and expenditure patterns may shift as well.

Compensation describes these counter-responses. It is not sabotage, and it is not failure. The system is not acting against itself. It is responding to changed conditions by adjusting variables that influence energy availability, energy use, storage, release, and visible output. These adjustments can make weight response less direct, less immediate, or less proportional than expected, but they remain part of regulation. Compensation is regulation under changed conditions.

Compensation is best understood as variable adjustment. When intake, expenditure, activity, sleep, stress, recovery, or energy availability changes, the system may respond through changes in hunger, satiety, cravings, fatigue, spontaneous movement, recovery allocation, expenditure patterns, storage access, fluid balance, and substrate handling. These responses do not always occur in the same combination or with the same intensity. A system under one set of conditions may respond primarily through appetite pressure. Another may respond through fatigue or reduced movement. Another may show more visible fluid change because recovery or glycogen dynamics are involved.

This means compensation is rarely a clean one-for-one offset. It may be partial, delayed, uneven, or context-dependent. It may reduce the visible effect of an input change without eliminating it. It may appear after a lag rather than immediately. It may occur in one domain while another domain continues moving in the original direction. The original change still matters, but it becomes only one moving variable inside a wider system response.

Reduced intake illustrates this clearly. A reduction in energy entering the system changes more than the intake side of the equation. It can alter perceived energy availability, which may influence hunger intensity, appetite timing, cravings, fatigue, spontaneous movement, recovery allocation, storage and release dynamics, and expenditure patterns. The system interprets lower availability in relation to current demand, prior intake, recovery state, stress load, activity, and adaptive history.

This does not mean reduced intake is irrelevant. It means reduced intake enters a responsive system. When availability changes, the system may adjust other variables that influence the final output. Hunger may rise because intake pressure has changed. Spontaneous movement may decline without deliberate intention. Fatigue may increase, altering the amount of energy used through ordinary motion. Recovery demands may compete more strongly for available resources. Storage access and release patterns may shift depending on signaling and prior conditions. The visible output may therefore be less direct than a static model would predict.

The same principle applies to increased activity. Activity changes energy use during movement, but the system response does not end when the movement stops. Increased or repeated activity may alter appetite pressure, fatigue, recovery demand, glycogen dynamics, fluid regulation, substrate use, spontaneous movement later in the day, and expenditure patterns elsewhere. The visible activity is only one part of the total response.

This does not mean activity is irrelevant. It means activity enters a broader regulatory context. Tissue stress may require repair. Glycogen use may affect water balance. Recovery demand may redirect energy and fluid. Fatigue may reduce later movement. Appetite pressure may shift because demand has increased. Expenditure may rise in one domain while another domain adjusts. The total effect of activity is therefore not limited to the activity itself; it includes the system's response to the demand created by that activity.

Compensation can move through several routes. Appetite is one route. When availability decreases or demand increases, hunger may rise, satiety may change, cravings may become more salient, or intake pressure may shift in timing. These signals are not moral events. They are part of the system's effort to regulate energy availability under changed conditions.

Fatigue is another route. Fatigue can reduce output, alter movement, and change how much energy is allocated toward nonessential activity. Spontaneous movement may shift without deliberate planning through changes in posture, fidgeting, walking, household motion, or general restlessness. These adjustments can be subtle, but they matter because expenditure is distributed across both visible and less visible movement.

Recovery allocation provides another route. When activity, stress, or reduced availability increases repair demand, energy and fluid may be directed toward restoration. This can influence visible weight through inflammation, fluid retention, glycogen replenishment, and tissue repair processes. Storage and release dynamics may also shift as the system manages current demand against available resources. Expenditure may change across domains rather than rising or falling as one uniform number. Fluid regulation can alter visible weight independently of longer-term tissue change, making the output appear inconsistent even when the system is responding coherently.

These routes often overlap rather than appearing separately. Appetite may rise at the same time fatigue reduces movement. Recovery demand may increase while fluid regulation changes visible weight. Expenditure may shift across domains while storage and release dynamics adjust to altered availability. This overlap is why compensation can be difficult to isolate from the outside. The visible output reflects the combined response, not a single route operating alone.

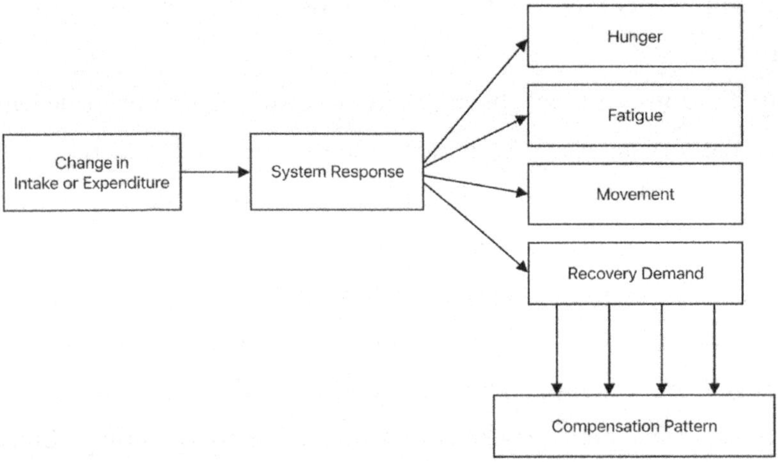

[Figure 10: Compensation Responses]

The figure represents one change leading to multiple possible counter-responses. A reduction in intake or increase in activity can trigger changes in appetite pressure, fatigue, spontaneous movement, recovery demand, expenditure patterns, storage and release, substrate handling, and fluid regulation. The original change remains real, but it is no longer the only variable moving inside the system.

Compensation makes weight change non-linear because several system variables can change together. A reduction in intake may produce one response initially, then another later as appetite pressure, fatigue, movement, recovery allocation, or expenditure patterns shift. Increased activity may produce an immediate expenditure change, followed by later changes in recovery demand, fluid balance, appetite, or spontaneous movement. The visible output may lag behind the original change because internal adjustment occurs first.

This also increases variability. Fluid regulation, glycogen dynamics, digestion, and recovery demand can shift while storage and release are also changing. The scale reports the net result of these moving parts, not the isolated effect of one input. Cause and effect can therefore appear blurred when compensation is ignored. The system may be responding in multiple domains while the visible output compresses those responses into one number.

Abrupt shifts can create stronger offsetting pressure because they change availability or demand quickly. A sudden reduction in intake may intensify appetite pressure, fatigue, or movement conservation more than a smaller or more predictable change. A sudden increase in activity may increase recovery demand, fluid shifts, glycogen turnover, or later movement compensation. The system responds not only to the direction of change, but also to its size, speed, and context.

Stable patterns may create less interpretive noise because the system has more predictable conditions to regulate around. When availability and demand are more consistent, appetite, movement, recovery, and fluid regulation may produce fewer abrupt counter-responses. This is not a prescription. It is a structural point: sudden changes often produce more visible regulatory pressure than conditions the system can anticipate and integrate with greater continuity.

Compensation does not erase energy balance. It changes how energy balance operates. Energy balance is not a pair of frozen numbers in which intake and expenditure remain static after one variable changes. If intake changes, expenditure-related variables may also change. If activity changes, appetite or spontaneous movement may also change. If recovery demand changes, fluid balance and expenditure patterns may shift.

Compensation does not violate energy balance; it changes the system variables inside it. Energy entering, energy used, energy stored, and energy released still constrain the system. But those quantities interact rather than remaining independent. Intake can influence appetite and expenditure. Activity can influence recovery and later movement. Stress and sleep can influence fluid regulation and energy allocation. Storage and release can shift in response to availability and demand. The balance remains real, but the variables inside it are dynamic.

This distinction prevents compensation from being misread as contradiction. A delayed response does not mean the system ignored the input. A smaller-than-expected response does not mean energy balance disappeared. A variable response does not mean the output is random. It means the system adjusted several connected processes while integrating the original change.

Compensation is one reason weight regulation cannot be interpreted through isolated inputs alone. A single change in intake or activity does not occur in a sealed chamber. It occurs inside a responsive system that may adjust appetite, fatigue, movement, recovery, storage and release, fluid regulation, and expenditure. Compensation makes the system dynamic, not contradictory. It does not violate energy balance; it changes the variables inside it.

Plateau Mechanism

A plateau is often misread because the visible output appears still. When the scale does not move much across an observed period, stillness can seem like an explanation in itself. The number appears unchanged, and that unchanged number can create the impression that nothing is happening beneath it. Because weight is visible as a single value, a stable value can be mistaken for a silent system.

That interpretation is too narrow. The scale only reports the final visible output. It does not show whether appetite pressure has shifted, whether expenditure has reorganized, whether spontaneous movement has changed, whether recovery demand is altering fluid balance, or whether storage and release dynamics are adjusting beneath the surface. A stable output does not prove internal inactivity. It only shows that the combined result of many processes has not changed enough to appear as a new visible direction.

A plateau is therefore an interpretation problem before it is anything else. The stillness of the number invites a conclusion that the system has stopped, but the system does not stop simply because the output holds steady. Energy continues to enter, be used, be stored, be released, and be distributed. Signals continue to coordinate availability and demand. Appetite, recovery, fluid regulation, adaptation, and compensation continue to operate. The question is not whether the system is active. The question is how that activity is combining into a temporarily stable result.

A plateau can be defined as a period of temporary equilibrium in visible output. Equilibrium does not mean nothing is moving. It means the movement of several variables is producing a stable combined effect. Intake may be changing slightly while expenditure shifts in response. Appetite pressure may be altering the input stream. Spontaneous movement may rise or fall without deliberate awareness. Recovery allocation may influence fluid retention. Storage and release may adjust to demand. Adaptation and compensation may change the relationship among these variables. The number remains stable because the net output is stable, not because the internal system is inactive.

This is the central correction: a plateau is not no activity. It is a form of system rebalancing. The visible output may hold steady while the system reorganizes the conditions that produce that output. The stillness belongs to the measurement, not necessarily to the underlying processes.

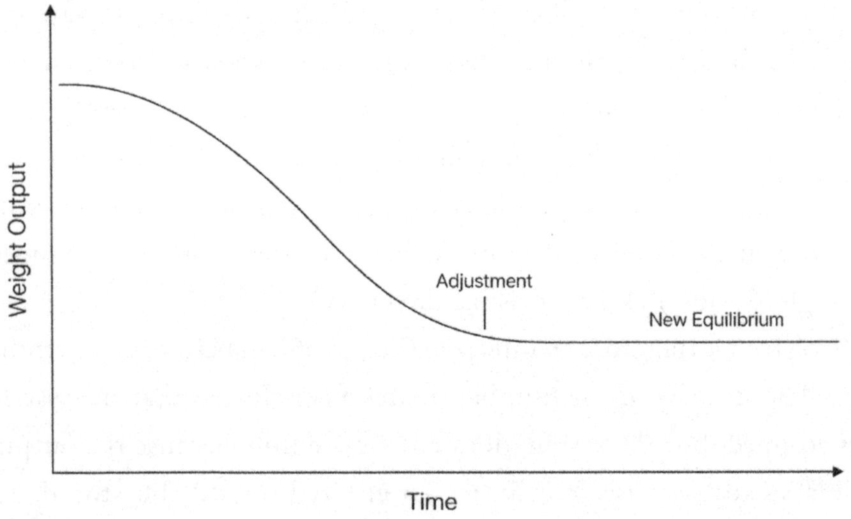

[Figure 11: Plateau as Temporary Equilibrium]

The figure represents multiple moving variables producing a stable visible output. Intake, expenditure, appetite, storage and release, recovery allocation, fluid regulation, adaptation, and compensation may all remain active while their combined effect produces little movement in the scale number.

A plateau is not necessarily failure. It does not automatically indicate lack of change, lack of effort, or system breakdown. It may reflect rebalancing after prior change. When one part of the system shifts, other parts may adjust around it. Compensation may alter appetite, fatigue, spontaneous movement, recovery demand, expenditure patterns, storage access, or fluid regulation. Adaptation may change the receiving state of the system so that the same inputs no longer produce the same visible output. These changes can produce a period of output stability.

This does not mean a plateau should be assigned a single universal meaning. It is not automatically beneficial, harmful, permanent, meaningless, or corrective. It is a signal that requires context. The same visible plateau can arise from different internal arrangements. One plateau may reflect fluid balance masking slower change. Another may reflect appetite and expenditure settling into a new relationship. Another may reflect recovery demand increasing while other variables move in the opposite direction. The visible stillness is real, but it is incomplete.

Internal rebalancing can occur through appetite. If the system perceives lower availability or increased demand, hunger and intake pressure may shift. Satiety may shorten or become less stable. Cravings may become more noticeable if prior conditions have changed the appetite signal environment. These changes can alter intake patterns subtly, without appearing as a distinct event. A plateau may emerge because appetite pressure has adjusted the input stream enough to balance other changes occurring elsewhere.

Expenditure can also reorganize across domains. Total energy use is not one fixed number. Resting function, spontaneous movement, formal activity, digestion, thermoregulation, recovery, and cellular maintenance all contribute. When conditions change, expenditure may shift in one domain while another remains stable or moves in the opposite direction. Spontaneous movement is especially important because it can change without deliberate intention. Small changes in posture, walking, fidgeting, household motion, and general physical restlessness can alter total expenditure while remaining nearly invisible to interpretation.

Storage and release dynamics add another layer. Stored energy may become more or less accessible depending on hormonal signaling, glycogen status, activity, sleep, stress, recovery, and prior intake. Glycogen and water can shift quickly, while longer-term storage patterns change more slowly and are harder to isolate. A plateau may occur when one storage-related process would lower visible weight while another process, such as fluid retention or glycogen replenishment, raises it. The scale reports the net result, not the opposing movements beneath it.

Recovery allocation can stabilize visible weight even while the system is active. Tissue repair, inflammation, immune activity, and cellular restoration can influence fluid balance. A system under recovery demand may retain more fluid while other variables shift toward lower mass. The result can be a stable visible output that masks internal movement. This is one reason plateaus cannot be interpreted from the scale alone. The number does not identify whether stability is coming from unchanged storage, altered fluid balance, recovery demand, or interacting processes.

Adaptation further complicates the visible plateau. Repeated conditions change the system's receiving state. A pattern that once produced one visible output may later produce another because appetite pressure, spontaneous movement, substrate handling, storage access, and expenditure patterns have recalibrated. Compensation may then stabilize the visible output by altering variables inside energy balance. The plateau becomes the visible expression of a new temporary arrangement, not a sign that regulation has stopped.

The system may stabilize at a new output level. A prior set of conditions may support one weight range for a period of time, then repeated patterns and internal adjustments may move the system toward another range. This new level reflects the interaction of intake, expenditure, storage, release, appetite, recovery, fluid regulation, adaptation, and compensation. It is not a final endpoint. It is a current equilibrium produced by the conditions operating at that time.

Temporary balance can persist until conditions change, until internal variables shift again, or until enough time reveals a new trend. A plateau may appear firm from the perspective of short-term observation, but biological systems remain dynamic. The output may stay stable while the system continues to adjust internally. Later movement can appear when the balance among variables changes. The plateau is a phase of output stability, not a permanent declaration about the system.

This is why interpretation requires trend, context, and time. A single unchanged reading is not a plateau. Several unchanged readings over a short period may still reflect ordinary variability, glycogen shifts, digestive contents, fluid balance, or recovery-related retention. Because weight is delayed and variable, short-term stillness has limited explanatory power. It may simply be one form of noise within a larger pattern.

A meaningful plateau becomes interpretable only across enough time to distinguish temporary stillness from sustained output stability. Context determines what that stability may represent. Prior intake patterns, activity, stress load, sleep, recovery state, appetite pressure, compensation, and adaptation all shape the meaning of the plateau. Without context, the plateau is only a visible fact: the number has not moved much. With context, it becomes information about the current balance of system variables.

Lag matters because the visible output may trail behind internal change. Variability matters because short-term movement or stillness may reflect fluid, glycogen, digestion, or recovery rather than longer-term direction. Adaptation matters because the system's response changes with repeated conditions. Compensation matters because one change can be offset by movement in other variables. Plateau sits at the intersection of these mechanisms. It is what output stability can look like when a delayed, variable, adaptive, compensating system temporarily balances itself.

A plateau should therefore be read as system information, not mysterious inactivity. It indicates that the current combination of variables is producing a stable visible result. It does not specify which variables are responsible. It does not prove that nothing is changing. It does not explain itself without time and context.

The central distinction remains the interpretive anchor. A plateau is not no activity. It is a form of system rebalancing.

Drift Mechanism

Drift is difficult to detect because it rarely presents itself as a single, identifiable event. There is no clear moment when the system announces that something has changed. Instead, the visible output begins to move gradually, often without a specific point of origin. The scale shifts slightly over time, and when that shift becomes noticeable, it can appear disconnected from any one cause.

This creates a common interpretive problem. When change is slow and lacks a clear trigger, it can feel unexplained. A person may look back and fail to identify a moment when intake increased, movement decreased, or routine shifted enough to account for the visible change. The absence of a single cause can make the change feel mysterious. But drift is not the absence of cause. It is the accumulation of many small causes that are individually difficult to detect.

Gradual change often becomes visible only after it has already been forming for some time. What appears to be a recent shift in output is often the delayed expression of earlier conditions. The system does not change suddenly at the moment the scale begins to move. The output becomes visible after enough time has passed for small differences to accumulate into a measurable result. Drift is therefore not an abrupt event but a process that becomes visible once its effects cross a threshold of detection.

Drift can be defined as gradual movement in visible output produced by small mismatches repeated across time. These mismatches may be subtle. They may not stand out in daily experience. Intake may shift slightly in quantity or timing. Movement may decrease in ways that are not consciously noticed. Sleep may become more irregular. Stress load may increase or remain elevated for longer periods. Recovery demand may accumulate. None of these changes needs to be dramatic to matter.

The mechanism does not depend on a specific direction. Drift can occur upward, downward, or toward a different range altogether. The defining feature is not whether weight increases or decreases, but that the change emerges slowly from repeated conditions. A system that is slightly offset from its prior balance, when exposed to the same offset repeatedly, will eventually produce a different output. The change appears gradual because each contributing difference is small, but the accumulation is not.

Small mismatches become visible when time amplifies them.

From the inside, drift can feel invisible because each individual change appears too small to matter. A slightly larger portion, a slightly shorter sleep period, a slightly more sedentary day, or a slightly elevated stress level may not register as meaningful. The system often absorbs these changes without producing an immediate visible response. Daily variation and short-term noise can easily mask their effects.

Lag further obscures detection. Weight does not update in real time with each small shift in intake or expenditure. The output reflects a combination of past and present conditions. This delay means that small mismatches may not produce immediate feedback. Without immediate feedback, the system's direction can change without being recognized at the time it is forming.

Variability adds another layer. Short-term fluctuations in fluid balance, glycogen, digestion, and recovery can create noise in the signal. This noise can conceal underlying direction. A small accumulating mismatch may be present, but the visible output may move up and down within a narrow range, making it difficult to distinguish trend from variation. The system may already be shifting, but the visible data does not yet reveal that shift clearly.

Over time, repetition becomes more important than magnitude. A small mismatch repeated consistently can have a larger effect than a large mismatch that occurs once. The system integrates repeated conditions. Each instance may seem negligible, but the cumulative effect is not. Drift emerges when these small differences are not isolated events but part of a repeated pattern.

The sources of small mismatch are varied and often interconnected. Intake can change in subtle ways. Portion sizes may increase or decrease slightly. Timing may shift, leading to different patterns of energy availability. Appetite signals may adjust in response to prior intake, stress, sleep, or routine. These changes may not be consciously tracked, yet they can alter the overall input pattern.

Movement can also shift without deliberate intention. Spontaneous activity—walking, standing, fidgeting, and general physical motion—can increase or decrease in response to fatigue, schedule, environment, or habit. These changes are often not experienced as decisions. They occur as part of the system's regulation. Over time, a slight reduction or increase in spontaneous movement can contribute to drift.

Sleep plays a role by influencing appetite, recovery, and energy availability. Small disruptions in sleep timing or duration can alter how the system regulates intake and expenditure. These disruptions may not be extreme. They may occur as minor variations in schedule or quality. Repeated over time, they can shift the signal environment in which appetite and energy use are coordinated.

Stress load can function similarly. A slightly elevated or prolonged stress state can influence appetite pressure, recovery allocation, fluid regulation, and expenditure patterns. Stress does not need to be acute or dramatic to matter. Persistent low-level changes can alter system behavior when they are sustained.

Aging introduces gradual changes in demand, recovery capacity, and system responsiveness. These changes are typically slow and continuous.

They do not present as a single event, but they can shift how the system handles intake, movement, and recovery over time. As these shifts accumulate, they can contribute to drift.

Schedule changes and environmental constraints can also create mismatch. A different work pattern, altered daily structure, or changes in routine can affect when and how energy is consumed and expended. These changes may not be perceived as significant disruptions, but they can alter the system's patterns of intake and movement.

Recovery debt can accumulate when demand exceeds recovery over time. The system may respond by adjusting appetite, fluid balance, and movement. These adjustments can contribute to gradual changes in visible output. Again, no single day may stand out. The effect emerges from repetition.

Storage and release dynamics participate as well. Energy is not only consumed and used immediately; it is stored and later accessed. Small differences in how energy is stored or released across repeated conditions can accumulate. Fluid regulation can amplify or obscure these changes in the short term, but over time the underlying direction becomes visible.

Each of these factors can contribute to small mismatches. None of them needs to be large. Their significance lies in their persistence.

Accumulation across time is the central mechanism of drift. A small mismatch may have little immediate effect because the system can absorb it. The difference between intake and expenditure, or between demand and recovery, may be small enough that it does not produce a noticeable change in output on a given day or week. However, if that mismatch repeats, the system does not reset between instances. Each repetition adds to the cumulative effect.

Time acts as an amplifier. It converts repeated small differences into a larger, visible change. The system integrates the mismatch across days, weeks, and months. What was initially too small to detect becomes detectable once enough instances have accumulated. The visible output begins to shift not because a large change occurred, but because many small changes have compounded.

Lag means that the visible shift often appears after the underlying direction has already been established. Variability means that the path toward that shift may not appear smooth or consistent. There may be periods of apparent stability or fluctuation that obscure the developing trend. Drift becomes recognizable when the accumulated effect exceeds the noise created by variability and delay.

This is why drift does not require a dramatic event. It does not depend on a clear cause that can be pointed to in isolation. It emerges from repeated small imbalances that are individually unremarkable but collectively meaningful. The system's behavior over time produces the output, not any single moment within that time.

Drift can occur in either direction. A system may drift upward when intake slightly exceeds expenditure or when movement decreases relative to prior patterns. It may drift downward when intake is slightly reduced, when demand increases, or when recovery conditions alter energy availability. It may also drift into a new range and stabilize there, reflecting a different balance of variables.

The direction is not the defining feature. The mechanism is neutral. It describes how gradual change emerges from accumulation. The same principles apply regardless of whether the output increases, decreases, or stabilizes at a new level. The system is responding to repeated conditions, not to a single event.

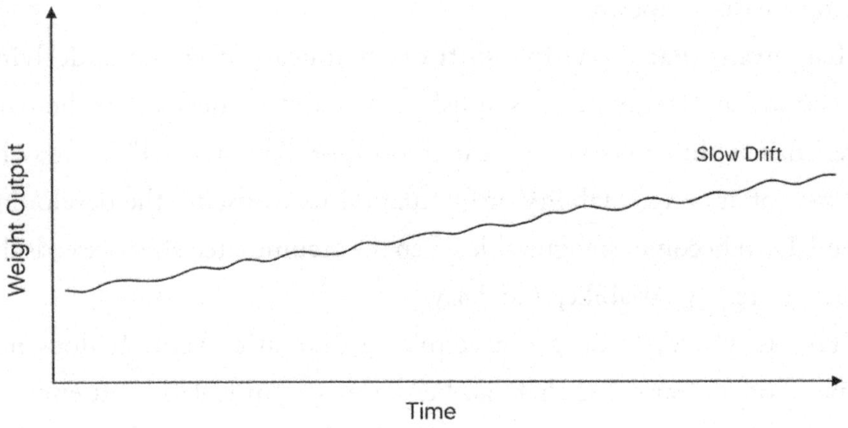

Small mismatches accumulate over time

[Figure 12: Slow Accumulation and Drift]

The figure illustrates how small repeated mismatches accumulate across time until the visible output changes enough to be recognized as drift. Each individual difference is small, but their repetition produces a larger effect.

Understanding drift requires an awareness of accumulation across time. Stability is not determined by a single day, a single input, or a single period of change. It is shaped by repeated patterns. A system that experiences consistent small mismatches will eventually produce a different output, even if no individual mismatch seems significant.

This does not mean that every small change will produce drift. The system is dynamic and can absorb variation. What matters is the pattern of repetition. When small differences persist, they become part of the system's operating conditions. Over time, these conditions shape the output.

Drift is therefore delayed evidence of accumulation. The visible change appears after the underlying process has already been in motion. What seems like an unexplained shift is often the result of many small, previously unnoticed factors that have been repeated long enough to matter.

The system did not change suddenly when the output became noticeable. The output became noticeable after time amplified the effect of small mismatches.

Small mismatches become visible when time amplifies them.

Glucose Interaction Mechanism

Glucose and weight are often discussed together, but they represent different types of information within the metabolic system. Glucose is a faster-moving signal. It changes across meals, fasting intervals, activity, stress, sleep, and recovery state. Weight is a slower accumulated output. It reflects storage, release, fluid regulation, tissue change, adaptation, compensation, and time. The relationship between them is real, but it is not interchangeable.

This distinction matters because it shapes how each should be interpreted. Glucose can move within hours. It can rise and fall in response to intake, demand, or internal signaling. Weight does not move in that way. It reflects the combined result of many processes operating across longer periods. A short-term signal cannot be read as a long-term outcome without losing context. Glucose provides information about current conditions. Weight provides information about accumulated conditions.

The connection between them lies in the fact that glucose participates in the system that produces weight. It does not define that system. It is one signal among many that help coordinate how energy is handled, routed, and made available. Weight is produced from the integration of those coordinated processes over time.

Glucose functions as an immediate signal of energy availability and fuel handling. When energy enters the system through intake, glucose can appear in circulation as part of that process. Its movement reflects that energy has become available for use or storage. When demand increases, glucose availability can shift to support that demand. When conditions change through stress or recovery, glucose patterns can also adjust.

This responsiveness makes glucose a useful indicator of current metabolic conditions. It can reflect how the system is handling recent input, how quickly energy is being made available, or how different states of demand are being met. Because it moves quickly, it can show changes that occur within the same day or even within a few hours. It is part of the system's short-term signaling layer.

However, this immediacy also means that glucose does not carry the same type of information as weight. It reflects what is happening now or very recently. It does not accumulate in the same way that weight does. A momentary shift in glucose does not represent the long-term balance of intake, expenditure, storage, and release. It represents a current state within that larger system.

Post-meal handling illustrates how glucose interacts with the processes that eventually contribute to weight. After intake, glucose movement is coordinated with hormonal signaling, particularly through mechanisms that regulate how energy is used, stored, or made available later. This coordination influences whether energy is directed toward immediate use, replenishment of short-term stores such as glycogen, or longer-term storage.

These processes are not controlled by glucose alone. Glucose participates as a signal within a coordinated network. Insulin and other signals help determine how energy is routed. Storage access and release dynamics influence how previously stored energy is used. Glycogen levels, activity, and recovery demand all interact with these signals. Glucose movement reflects part of this coordination, but it does not define the entire process.

This is why glucose should be understood as part of routing and signaling rather than as a single cause. It helps indicate how energy is being handled in the short term. It interacts with the processes that determine whether energy is used immediately or stored for later. But those processes are shaped by multiple variables, including prior conditions, demand, hormonal coordination, and system state.

Glucose patterns can also contribute to the clarity of regulation. When glucose movement is relatively stable and consistent, the system may be operating in a way that reduces signal noise. Energy availability may be easier to coordinate because signals are not shifting abruptly or unpredictably. Appetite signals, storage access, and energy use may align more smoothly under these conditions.

This does not imply a direct outcome for weight. Stable glucose patterns do not guarantee a specific direction of change in weight, nor do they determine body composition. They are part of a signaling environment that may support clearer coordination. When signals are more consistent, the system may be able to align energy availability with demand more efficiently. This can influence how the system behaves, but it does not replace the broader mechanisms that produce weight over time.

The relationship between glucose stability and system clarity is therefore indirect. Glucose can reduce or increase noise within the signaling environment. That environment includes appetite regulation, hormonal coordination, and energy routing. These factors interact with intake, expenditure, storage, and recovery. The outcome that appears as weight reflects the combined effect of all these processes, not the glucose pattern alone.

This leads to an important limitation: weight cannot be interpreted from glucose alone. Glucose is one signal within a larger system. Weight reflects the integration of that system across time. A glucose pattern may indicate how energy is being handled in the short term, but it does not capture the full range of variables that determine long-term output.

Weight reflects intake volume, expenditure across multiple domains, storage and release dynamics, glycogen and water shifts, sodium and fluid regulation, recovery demand, hormonal coordination, appetite patterns, sleep, stress, adaptation, compensation, plateau, drift, and time. Each of these factors contributes to the final output. Glucose participates in some of these interactions, but it does not encompass them.

For example, a given glucose pattern may appear similar across different conditions, yet the underlying system may be operating differently. One situation may involve higher recovery demand and fluid retention, while another may involve lower spontaneous movement and different storage dynamics. The glucose signal may not distinguish these differences clearly, but the weight outcome may reflect them over time.

Similarly, weight can change while glucose patterns remain relatively stable. A gradual shift in intake, movement, or recovery may accumulate without producing a dramatic change in short-term glucose signals. The output may move over weeks or months even if daily glucose variation appears consistent. This reflects the difference between short-term signaling and long-term accumulation.

The difference in time scale is central to understanding the relationship. Glucose operates on a short time scale. It responds quickly to intake, demand, and internal signals. Weight operates on a longer time scale. It reflects accumulated interactions across days, weeks, and months. These time scales do not align in a simple way.

A change in glucose within a day does not translate directly into a change in weight. The system integrates many such signals before producing a visible output. The lag between input, signaling, and output means that short-term changes can be misleading if interpreted as immediate predictors of long-term outcomes. Glucose can show that something has changed in the present. Weight shows what has accumulated across time.

This difference prevents overinterpretation. A short-term glucose pattern cannot fully explain a long-term weight trend. It can provide context, but it cannot replace the broader system analysis. The same glucose pattern may correspond to different weight outcomes depending on intake, expenditure, storage, recovery, and adaptation. The system's history and current state determine how signals are translated into output.

Glucose should therefore be placed within the system rather than above it. It matters because it reflects energy availability and handling. It interacts with hormonal coordination, storage access, and fuel routing. It can influence and be influenced by appetite, activity, stress, and recovery. But it does not operate in isolation, and it does not define the system's output on its own.

Weight is produced by the accumulation of interactions among many variables. Glucose is one of the signals that participates in those interactions. Its value lies in what it reveals about current conditions, not in its ability to predict or determine long-term outcomes by itself.

Understanding this distinction allows glucose to be interpreted without assigning it an outsized role. It can be seen as part of the system's communication layer. It provides information about how energy is being handled in the moment. That information can be useful in understanding system behavior, but it must be integrated with other variables to make sense of long-term patterns.

The system does not operate through a single signal. It operates through coordinated interactions. Glucose is one of the signals that contributes to that coordination. Weight is the output that reflects the result of those interactions over time.

Glucose can help illuminate the processes that contribute to weight, but it cannot replace them. Weight cannot be reduced to a single signal without losing the complexity that defines it.

Glucose is a signal within the system. Weight is an accumulated output of the system.

Fasting Interaction Mechanism

Fasting is often discussed as if it directly produces a specific outcome, but within a systems framework it is more accurately understood as a change in conditions. It alters when energy enters the system and creates periods in which incoming energy is absent. This change in timing and availability modifies how the system must regulate energy, but it does not command a particular result. The system continues to operate through storage and release, hormonal coordination, appetite signaling, recovery allocation, and prior state. Fasting changes the environment in which these processes occur. It does not determine their final output.

This distinction matters because it prevents a collapse of explanation into a single variable. When fasting is treated as a direct cause of weight change, the rest of the system disappears from the interpretation. In practice, the system remains active and responsive. The absence of input does not suspend regulation. It shifts the conditions under which regulation continues.

Fasting changes input timing. When intake is delayed, shortened, clustered, or absent for a period, the system receives energy under a different temporal structure. Instead of frequent or continuous input, there are intervals where incoming energy is not present. This alters how the system organizes energy availability across time. Glucose patterns adjust to reflect these intervals. Insulin signaling follows a different rhythm. Fuel routing must account for the absence of immediate input. Hunger signals may align with new timing patterns or remain influenced by prior patterns.

These timing changes do not carry inherent direction. They do not prescribe a specific pattern of storage or release. They require the system to coordinate energy across a different schedule. The same total intake distributed differently across time can produce different internal conditions, but those conditions still interact with the rest of the system. Timing modifies the structure of input, not the totality of response.

Input absence creates a different metabolic environment. During a fasting interval, the system relies more on stored energy and regulated release rather than immediate intake. Glycogen becomes a more prominent short-term buffer. Fatty acid availability may increase as the system draws on longer-term stores. Glucose availability shifts as intake is no longer supplying immediate input. Hormonal signals adjust to coordinate these changes, influencing how energy is accessed and distributed.

These changes are part of normal system function. The system is designed to operate across periods of both input and absence. The presence of a fasting interval does not introduce a new mechanism; it shifts the balance among existing ones. Storage and release dynamics become more visible during absence because the system must rely on them more directly. Hunger signaling may shift as the system responds to perceived availability. Energy use continues, supported by internal reserves rather than incoming input.

It is important to keep these changes in context. Altered fuel use during a fasting interval does not automatically translate into a long-term change in weight. The system may use stored energy during absence, but the overall output depends on how intake, expenditure, storage, and release interact across a longer horizon. A period of absence is one part of that interaction, not the entire explanation.

Even when internal conditions shift quickly during fasting, weight remains a delayed output. The system may change fuel use, glycogen levels, fluid balance, and hormonal signaling within hours, but the scale does not update in real time to reflect these changes in a simple way. Short-term weight movement may reflect changes in glycogen-associated water, digestive contents, or fluid regulation rather than longer-term shifts in stored energy.

This delay creates an interpretive gap. The internal state can change before the visible output becomes clear. A fasting interval may alter how energy is being handled, but the scale may not immediately reflect those changes, or it may reflect them in a way that is influenced by short-term variables. The visible number can move for reasons that are not directly tied to longer-term storage or release. This reinforces the need to separate short-term signal changes from accumulated output.

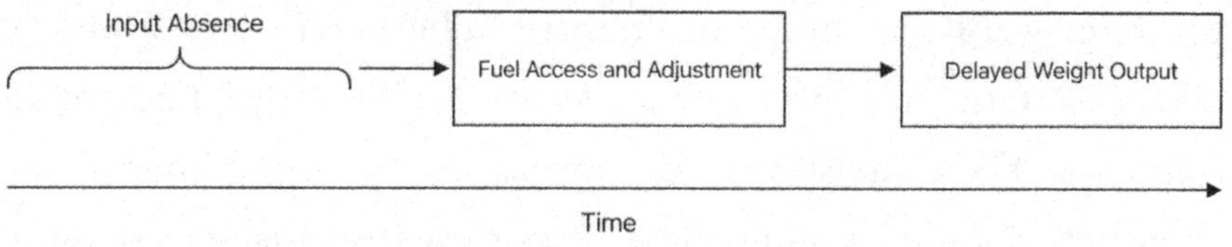

[Figure 13: Fasting Input Absence and Delayed Output]

The figure represents fasting as a period of input absence that changes internal conditions before any long-term weight output becomes clear. It illustrates how fuel availability, signaling, and storage dynamics can shift within the interval, while the visible output remains delayed and influenced by multiple interacting variables.

The system's response to fasting depends on prior state. The same fasting interval does not enter an empty system. It enters a system shaped by recent intake patterns, glycogen status, sleep, stress load, recovery demand, activity, appetite rhythms, and adaptive history. A system that has recently received consistent intake may experience a fasting interval differently from one that has been under prolonged variability or constraint. A system that is well recovered may coordinate energy availability differently from one under cumulative strain.

These differences do not imply that one response is correct and another is not. They reflect the system's continuity. The receiving state matters because it shapes how signals are interpreted and how energy is routed. Hunger intensity, perceived energy availability, and compensation pressure can all vary depending on prior conditions. The same absence of input can be experienced as relatively neutral in one context and more demanding in another.

Appetite and compensation are part of this response. Input absence can influence hunger signals during the fasting interval and after it. Appetite pressure may shift in timing or intensity. The system may adjust later intake, spontaneous movement, or recovery allocation in response to the absence. These adjustments do not negate the fasting interval. They demonstrate that the system remains responsive to changes in conditions.

Compensation can appear through multiple routes. Hunger may increase during or after the interval. Fatigue may influence movement or energy use. Spontaneous activity may shift without deliberate awareness. Recovery demand may alter fluid balance or energy allocation. These responses are not uniform, and they do not occur in the same way in every situation. They illustrate that fasting is received by a system that adjusts multiple variables at once.

This interaction is why fasting cannot be treated as a guaranteed driver of a specific outcome. The absence of input may create conditions that support certain patterns of energy use, but the system can respond by adjusting other variables. The final output reflects the combined effect of these adjustments across time.

Fasting can function as a structural change within the system. By altering input timing, it can change how frequently energy enters the system and how energy availability is distributed across the day or week. This structural change may simplify patterns of intake for some systems. It may reduce the frequency of feeding events or create clearer intervals between them. It may alter how hunger signals are experienced or how energy availability is coordinated.

These structural effects do not guarantee a particular direction of change. They modify the environment in which the system operates. For some systems, this may align with existing patterns in a way that produces a stable or shifting output. For others, the response may be different. The same structural change can produce different outcomes depending on how it interacts with intake amount, expenditure, storage, release, appetite, recovery, sleep, stress, and adaptation.

The broader system determines the output. Fasting interacts with intake volume, not just timing. It interacts with expenditure across multiple domains. It interacts with storage and release dynamics, which determine how energy is accessed during absence. It interacts with glucose signaling and hormonal coordination, which influence routing and availability. It interacts with appetite, which shapes intake pressure before and after the interval. It interacts with sleep and stress, which influence recovery and signaling. It interacts with adaptation and compensation, which change how the system responds to repeated conditions.

Weight is produced by this entire network of interactions across time. Fasting is one condition within that network. It does not replace the rest of the system. It does not override the variables that determine how energy is accumulated, stored, released, and reflected in the output.

This perspective removes the need to assign fasting a fixed role. It is neither a guaranteed driver of change nor an irrelevant variable. It is a condition that alters timing and availability. Its effect depends on how the system receives and responds to that condition. The outcome cannot be read from the fasting interval alone because the interval is only one part of a larger system.

The relationship between fasting and weight stability is therefore indirect. Fasting changes the context in which energy is managed. It can influence signals and processes that contribute to weight over time. But the weight output emerges from accumulated interactions, not from the presence or absence of a single condition.

Fasting changes conditions; it does not guarantee a specific weight output.

Flexibility Interaction Mechanism

Metabolic flexibility is often misunderstood when it is treated as a direct mechanism of weight change. In that frame, flexibility becomes a promise: a system that shifts fuels well is assumed to produce a specific weight outcome. That interpretation narrows the concept too quickly. Metabolic flexibility is not a weight-loss mechanism by itself. It is a system capacity.

This misreading is not accidental. Flexibility involves glucose use, fat use, storage, and release—processes that are closely associated with energy balance and body mass. Because these processes are visible in moment-to-moment physiology, it becomes easy to assume that changing fuel use in the present moment directly determines long-term weight. But fuel use in a given interval is not the same as accumulated change in stored mass. A system may rely more heavily on one fuel during a particular period without that period determining the long-term output. The distinction between momentary fuel selection and accumulated storage across time is what separates flexibility from weight as an outcome.

At the simplest level, metabolic flexibility describes the ability to shift among glucose use, fat use, storage, and release depending on conditions. The body does not operate in one fuel state at all times. It moves across fed-state handling, fasting-state reliance, activity-related demand, rest, recovery, and changing availability. These states overlap. They are not rigid compartments. They are patterns of energy handling shaped by intake, timing, demand, hormonal coordination, recovery, and prior conditions.

This capacity matters because weight regulation occurs inside a changing energy environment. Energy availability is not constant. Intake arrives in episodes. Demand rises and falls. Activity changes substrate use. Sleep and stress alter signaling. Recovery redirects resources. A flexible system can shift among available fuels and stored fuels as conditions change. That shifting can influence the environment in which weight stability is produced, but it does not determine weight in isolation.

Glucose use and fat use are often presented as opposing states, but in a functioning system they are better understood as coordinated options. The body can use incoming glucose when it is available, store energy when availability exceeds immediate demand, access stored energy when input is absent, and rely more heavily on different substrates as conditions shift. These transitions are not declarations of success or failure. They are forms of allocation.

Across a single day, the system may move through multiple overlapping emphases rather than a single dominant mode. After intake, glucose handling may be more prominent as incoming fuel is processed and distributed. As time passes without additional input, reliance on stored energy may increase. During activity, demand may shift toward more immediate fuel availability, while recovery periods may redirect energy toward repair and restoration. These are not discrete switches that lock the body into one identity. They are adjustments within a continuous process of energy management.

The body does not need to be categorized as "glucose-based" or "fat-based" in any fixed sense. It continuously coordinates available fuel, stored fuel, demand, and timing. Metabolic flexibility describes how effectively these shifts occur in response to changing conditions. It does not assign the system a permanent fuel identity.

Energy availability is one of the main places flexibility becomes relevant. When the system can shift more smoothly between incoming fuel and stored fuel, availability may be easier to coordinate across changing conditions. Transitions between feeding and fasting, rest and activity, input and absence, demand and recovery may create less disruption when the system can access and route energy appropriately. This is not an outcome promise. It is a description of coordination.

The connection to fasting is direct but limited. During input absence, the system relies more on stored energy and regulated release. Metabolic flexibility may influence how that transition is handled, how available energy is maintained, and how hunger or fatigue emerges during the interval. But the fasting interval still enters a broader system shaped by prior intake, glycogen status, sleep, stress, recovery demand, activity, and adaptation. Flexibility can affect the experience and coordination of input absence without guaranteeing a specific weight output.

During these intervals, the system must maintain function while incoming energy is delayed. The ease or strain of that process depends on more than the presence or absence of intake. Storage access, glycogen status, hormonal coordination, sleep quality, stress load, recovery demand, and prior intake patterns all influence how the system manages the absence of new input. These factors can shape hunger, fatigue, attention, and perceived energy availability during the interval. The same fasting period may therefore feel stable in one context and strained in another, not because the interval itself has changed, but because the system receiving it has.

Fuel selection can also influence hunger, fatigue, and daily function. If energy availability becomes unstable during transitions, hunger pressure may become more noticeable. Fatigue may appear when demand and availability do not align cleanly. If transitions are smoother, changes in input timing or activity demand may produce less disruption in the signal environment. These effects remain contextual. They do not promise appetite control, performance change, or a specific body outcome.

This is where flexibility interacts with appetite regulation. Appetite signals are shaped partly by perceived energy availability. If the system has difficulty coordinating access to energy during changing conditions, hunger or cravings may become more prominent. If energy availability is more stable, appetite signals may be less noisy. But appetite is still shaped by sleep, stress, prior intake, environment, routine, and recovery. Flexibility participates in the signal environment; it does not replace it.

The relationship between flexibility, storage, and release is equally important. Storage and release are often interpreted as opposing outcomes, but within the system they are complementary functions. Storage allows energy to be held for later use when availability exceeds immediate demand. Release allows that stored energy to support function when incoming energy is lower or demand rises. Both processes are necessary. Neither represents a system failure.

Metabolic flexibility affects how smoothly the system moves between these functions. A system that can coordinate storage and release across changing conditions may experience smoother transitions in energy availability. But the presence of storage in one moment or release in another does not determine weight by itself. Weight stability depends on how these processes balance across time, not on whether one process is active at a single point.

Yet weight is not a direct measure of flexibility. Two systems may show similar weight outputs while differing substantially in glucose handling, fuel switching, appetite pressure, fasting tolerance, fatigue, storage access, and response to input absence. The same visible output can be produced by different internal arrangements. Weight compresses these differences into a single number, and that compression removes detail.

The reverse is also true. Changes in flexibility may not immediately appear as changes in weight. A system may handle transitions differently—experiencing different patterns of energy availability, hunger, or fatigue—while the scale remains stable because intake, expenditure, fluid regulation, recovery demand, or compensation are also shifting.

Flexibility can change the internal environment without immediately changing the visible output.

This makes weight an unreliable proxy for flexibility. A stable weight does not confirm stable fuel handling, and a changing weight does not isolate flexibility as the cause. Weight may shift because of fluid balance, intake volume, recovery demand, reduced movement, sleep disruption, or accumulated drift. These factors can move independently of changes in fuel-switching capacity.

Over longer time horizons, flexibility may contribute to how the system navigates changing conditions, but even then it remains one component among many. It interacts with intake patterns, activity levels, sleep, stress, recovery, hormonal coordination, adaptation, and compensation. The visible output reflects the combined effect of these variables, not the influence of flexibility alone.

This prevents an important overinterpretation. Flexibility may influence the conditions around energy handling, but weight remains a long-term accumulated output. It reflects intake, expenditure, storage, release, appetite, hormonal coordination, sleep, stress, recovery, adaptation, compensation, plateau, drift, and time. No single capacity, including flexibility, explains the whole output.

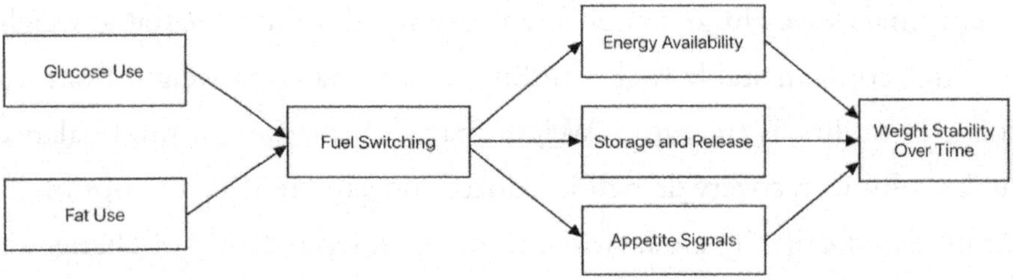

[Figure 14: Fuel Switching, Storage, and Release]

The figure represents glucose use, fat use, storage, and release as interacting system states rather than separate weight outcomes. The system moves among these states depending on availability, demand, timing, recovery, and prior conditions.

Metabolic flexibility is best understood as a surrounding condition of weight regulation. It shapes how the system handles transitions, how energy availability is maintained, how hunger and fatigue may appear, and how storage and release are coordinated. These effects matter because weight is produced inside that environment. But the environment is not the output itself.

The visible weight output still depends on accumulated conditions across time. Fuel switching may influence the path, but the final signal reflects the whole system. Metabolic flexibility affects the conditions around weight regulation, not weight in isolation.

Trend Mechanism

A single weight reading is easy to overinterpret because it is immediate, visible, and discrete. It presents itself as a clear statement: a number that appears to describe the current state of the system. That clarity is misleading. The number is real, but its meaning is not self-contained. It is one point within a system that is delayed, variable, and influenced by multiple interacting processes.

An isolated measurement often feels more meaningful than it is because it is specific. It can be seen, compared, and remembered. But the system that produces it is not momentary. It is continuous. A single reading may reflect fluid balance, glycogen status, digestive contents, recovery demand, sodium, sleep disruption, stress, or timing effects rather than the longer direction of the system. The visible point is precise, but the interpretation attached to it may not be.

This creates a separation between visibility and interpretive value. What is seen is not always what is most informative. The most visible signal is not necessarily the most accurate representation of the system's direction. That distinction becomes clearer when weight is understood not as a momentary statement, but as an output produced across time.

Trend provides the frame that resolves this mismatch. It is the pattern that emerges when individual measurements are placed across a longer horizon. A trend does not eliminate noise, but it reduces the influence of any single noisy point. It allows the observer to see whether the system is generally stable, drifting, rising, falling, or fluctuating around a range.

The individual readings remain, but their meaning changes when they are understood as part of a sequence rather than as isolated events.

A point is not a pattern.

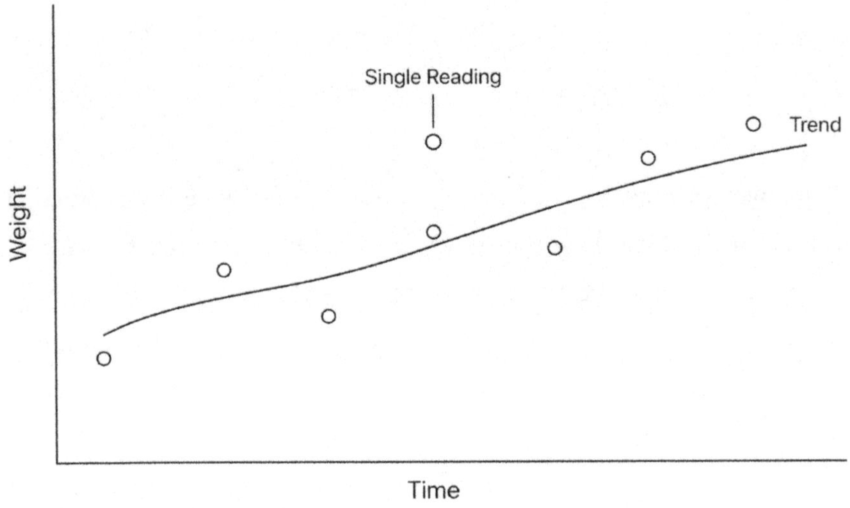

[Figure 15: Point Versus Pattern]

The figure shows how individual points can appear inconsistent or misleading when viewed alone, while the broader pattern reveals the direction of the system. The same set of measurements can suggest instability at the level of single readings and coherence at the level of trend.

Short-term noise is one reason isolated readings can mislead. Weight can shift from one day to the next because of changes in fluid distribution, glycogen storage, digestive contents, inflammatory response, sodium intake, sleep variation, stress signaling, or the timing of measurement. These shifts can be substantial enough to appear meaningful, even when they do not reflect a change in longer-term storage or release.

This noise can obscure direction in two ways. It can create the appearance of movement when the underlying pattern is stable, and it can create the appearance of stability when a slower trend is forming. A series of fluctuating readings may conceal a gradual upward or downward movement, while a temporary plateau in visible output may hide internal adjustments that have not yet become apparent in the pattern. Noise does not remove information, but it complicates its interpretation.

The role of variability in this process is not to distort the system, but to reflect the multiple inputs that influence the output. Weight is not a single-variable signal. It responds to a combination of fluid shifts, substrate availability, storage and release dynamics, and recovery processes. These influences do not move in perfect alignment, and their interaction produces variability. Trend allows that variability to be contextualized rather than taken at face value.

Lag adds another layer to this interpretive challenge. Weight does not respond immediately to changes in intake, expenditure, or internal conditions. The visible output may trail behind the processes that generate it. A system may already be changing before the pattern becomes clear, and a single reading may reflect conditions that occurred earlier rather than the present state.

This delay means that the meaning of a reading cannot be understood in isolation from time. A change in intake or activity may not appear immediately in the output, and a visible change may represent accumulated effects rather than recent inputs. Without a longer horizon, it becomes difficult to distinguish between immediate noise, delayed response, and emerging trend.

Trend helps resolve this by placing readings across enough time to reveal accumulated direction. It allows the observer to see whether the system is converging toward a new state, maintaining stability, or drifting gradually. The individual points remain variable, but their sequence reveals the underlying pattern.

Longer horizons are more informative because weight reflects accumulated system behavior. The processes that influence weight—intake patterns, movement patterns, recovery demand, sleep, stress, adaptation, compensation, plateau formation, drift, glucose handling, fasting structure, and metabolic flexibility—operate across time. They do not express themselves fully in a single moment.

When readings are viewed over a longer period, these processes begin to align into a pattern. Repeated conditions produce consistent effects, and those effects become visible as trend. A gradual increase may reflect accumulated mismatch. A stable range may reflect balanced inputs and outputs. A plateau may indicate temporary equilibrium among interacting variables. These interpretations are not available from a single reading because the processes that produce them require time to manifest.

This does not mean that individual readings are irrelevant. Each point is part of the pattern. But the meaning of the point depends on its position within the sequence. A single increase or decrease does not define the direction of the system. It becomes meaningful when it is placed alongside other readings and evaluated within the broader context.

The shift from event reaction to pattern recognition follows from this understanding. Event reaction treats each reading as an explanation. A change in the number is interpreted as a direct reflection of recent behavior or input. Pattern recognition asks a different question: whether the reading belongs to noise, lag, fluctuation, plateau, drift, or a broader directional change.

This shift is not about ignoring the data. It is about changing the level of interpretation. The focus moves from individual events to the structure that connects them. The reading is still observed, but it is not assigned meaning until it is understood within the pattern. This reduces the likelihood of misinterpreting noise as direction or mistaking temporary variation for system change.

Trend also provides information about stability. A stable trend does not indicate inactivity. It may indicate that the system is maintaining output within a range. This can occur when intake, expenditure, storage, release, appetite, recovery, and other variables are balanced in a way that produces consistent output. The system may still be active beneath the surface, but the visible signal remains within a defined range.

A noisy but range-bound pattern can indicate a stable operating zone. The individual readings may fluctuate, but the overall pattern remains consistent. This is different from drift, where small mismatches accumulate and gradually shift the output over time. It is also different from a plateau, where variables temporarily balance at a new level. Trend allows these distinctions to become visible.

A gradual upward or downward trend may indicate drift. A flat section may indicate a plateau. A fluctuating pattern around a stable range may indicate maintained equilibrium. These interpretations require a sequence of readings because they depend on how the system behaves across time, not on the value of any single point.

Trend does not eliminate uncertainty, but it reduces interpretive error. It does not make the system simple, but it makes the structure of the system more visible. It provides a frame in which noise, lag, variability, and accumulation can be understood together rather than in isolation.

This is why a longer horizon is necessary for interpreting weight. The system that produces weight operates continuously, and its output reflects that continuity. A single reading captures only a fragment of that process. The pattern that emerges across multiple readings captures more of the system's behavior.

Weight becomes more interpretable when readings are understood as part of a larger pattern. The visible point carries information, but the pattern carries context. Without context, the point can be misleading. With context, the same point can become meaningful.

The distinction is not between accuracy and inaccuracy, but between completeness and incompleteness. A single reading is accurate as a measurement, but incomplete as an interpretation. A trend provides a more complete view because it incorporates time, variability, and accumulation.

The system does not produce isolated points. It produces a continuous output that is sampled at discrete moments. Those samples only become informative when they are connected. Trend is the structure that connects them.

A point is not a pattern.

Consistency Mechanism

Consistency is often framed as a behavioral standard—something to achieve through discipline, repetition, or control. In that framing, it becomes a demand placed on the individual rather than a condition within the system. That interpretation obscures its role in understanding weight. In the context of weight stability, consistency is better understood as an interpretive condition.

When the inputs and surrounding conditions that shape weight change constantly, the output becomes more difficult to read. The system is still producing a result, but that result reflects multiple shifting influences at once. A reading taken under those circumstances may be accurate, but its meaning is harder to isolate. When patterns are more stable, the system's response becomes easier to observe across time. The output does not become simpler, but the relationship between input and output becomes clearer.

This distinction separates consistency from control. Consistency does not command the system to produce a specific outcome. It does not eliminate variability, remove delay, or override adaptation and compensation. What it does is reduce random variation in the conditions producing the output. In doing so, it improves the clarity of what the output represents.

Consistency makes output easier to interpret; it does not create immediate control.

Inconsistent inputs and conditions can create outputs that appear erratic even when the system is functioning normally. Intake timing may shift from one day to the next. Activity demand may vary with schedule, environment, or energy levels. Sleep may be stable one night and disrupted the next. Stress may rise and fall unpredictably. Recovery demand may change with workload or health status. Fluid balance, sodium exposure, and appetite rhythms may all fluctuate within short periods.

Each of these variables can influence weight independently, but their combined effect is what produces the visible output. When many of them change at once, the system is responding to multiple inputs simultaneously. The resulting pattern may appear inconsistent, not because the system lacks structure, but because the conditions producing the output are themselves unstable. The reading reflects this mixture rather than a single identifiable influence.

This does not make variation a problem. Variation is inherent to biological systems. The system is designed to respond to changing conditions. The difficulty arises when variation is interpreted without context. When inputs shift frequently and unpredictably, it becomes harder to determine whether a change in output reflects noise, lag, adaptation, compensation, or an emerging trend. The system remains coherent, but the signal becomes more difficult to read.

Stable patterns reduce this interpretive noise. When conditions are more consistent across time, fewer variables are shifting unpredictably at the same moment. The system's response can still be complex, but the number of competing influences is lower. This makes it easier to observe how the system behaves under those conditions.

A change in output observed under relatively stable conditions may be easier to interpret because it is less likely to be obscured by unrelated fluctuations. If intake timing, movement demand, sleep, and recovery state are not shifting dramatically, then changes in weight may be more clearly associated with accumulated system behavior rather than short-term variation. This does not isolate cause, but it reduces the number of simultaneous explanations.

Consistency, in this sense, is not about holding every variable constant. It is about reducing random variation enough for patterns to become visible. Biological systems are not static. They do not operate under perfectly controlled conditions. Normal variation remains present even in relatively stable patterns. The goal is not elimination of variation, but reduction of unpredictability.

This is where consistency must be distinguished from rigidity. Rigidity implies fixed inputs, repeated without variation, as if the system requires identical conditions to function properly. That interpretation misrepresents both the system and the role of consistency. Systems can tolerate and respond to variation. They are built to adapt. Consistency does not require sameness at every moment. It requires enough stability across time for patterns to emerge.

A system can be consistent without being rigid. Intake can vary within a pattern. Activity can shift within a range. Sleep and stress can fluctuate while still maintaining overall structure. Consistency exists when these variations occur within a recognizable pattern rather than as unrelated, unpredictable changes. The distinction is not between change and no change, but between structured variation and random variation.

This distinction matters because interpretation depends on pattern recognition. When variation is structured, the output can be read as part of a pattern. When variation is random, the output becomes harder to place within any pattern. The same numerical reading can carry different meaning depending on whether it appears within a stable pattern or within a highly variable one.

Signal clarity is the central effect of consistency. The output becomes easier to interpret when there is less random variation in the inputs and conditions producing it. This clarity does not simplify the system, but it reduces the number of competing influences that must be considered at once. It allows distinctions to become more visible.

Under more stable conditions, it becomes easier to distinguish noise from pattern. Short-term fluctuations can be recognized as variability rather than as directional change. Lag can be identified as delayed response rather than immediate effect. A plateau can be recognized as temporary equilibrium rather than stagnation. Drift can be seen as gradual accumulation rather than sudden shift. Stability itself can be identified as maintained balance rather than inactivity.

This connects directly to trend. Trend reveals pattern across time, but the clarity of that pattern depends partly on the stability of the conditions producing it. When conditions shift constantly, the trend may be more difficult to interpret because it reflects multiple overlapping influences. When conditions are more stable, the trend may more clearly reflect accumulated system behavior. The pattern is still shaped by lag, variability, adaptation, and compensation, but it is less obscured by unrelated fluctuations.

Consistency therefore supports interpretation rather than outcome. It does not determine the direction of the trend. It makes the direction more visible. The system still responds according to its internal processes. Consistency does not override those processes. It reduces the noise surrounding them.

This is particularly important because weight remains a delayed output. Even under stable conditions, the system may take time to reveal its response. A consistent pattern does not produce immediate certainty. It produces delayed clarity. The system continues to operate with lag, and the visible output continues to reflect accumulated conditions rather than immediate inputs.

Adaptation and compensation also remain active under stable conditions. The system may adjust its response over time, altering appetite pressure, expenditure patterns, spontaneous movement, recovery allocation, and storage dynamics. These adjustments can change the relationship between input and output even when inputs appear stable. Consistency does not prevent these processes. It allows them to be observed more clearly.

This reinforces the distinction between interpretation and control. Consistency does not provide command over the system. It does not ensure a particular outcome. It does not eliminate delay, variability, or adaptive response. It improves the ability to understand what the system is doing across time.

When inputs and conditions vary widely, it becomes difficult to determine what the system is responding to. A change in output may coincide with multiple changes in input, making interpretation uncertain. When conditions are more stable, the relationship between pattern and output becomes easier to follow. The system is not simplified, but its behavior becomes more legible.

This legibility is what consistency provides. It is not a behavioral requirement. It is a structural property of the system's operating environment. When variation is reduced, the signal becomes clearer. When variation is high, the signal becomes more difficult to interpret.

This does not imply that more consistency always produces better outcomes. It implies that more consistency produces clearer information about the outcomes that are occurring. The distinction is important. The goal is not to produce a specific result, but to understand the result that is being produced.

In this way, consistency contributes to long-term stability not by controlling the system, but by clarifying it. It allows the observer to see how repeated conditions shape the output across time. It reduces the likelihood of misinterpreting noise as direction or mistaking temporary variation for meaningful change.

The system remains dynamic, responsive, and influenced by multiple interacting variables. Consistency does not remove that complexity. It provides a clearer view of it.

Consistency makes output easier to interpret; it does not create immediate control.

Outcome Stability Mechanism

Weight is visible, measurable, and easy to isolate. It appears as a single number, which makes it seem more complete than it is. The number can be recorded, compared, and followed across time, but its visibility does not make it self-explanatory. Weight is downstream of the system that produces it. It reflects accumulated regulation across intake, expenditure, storage, release, appetite, hormonal coordination, glucose handling, recovery, adaptation, compensation, trend, consistency, and time.

This does not make weight meaningless. A downstream signal can still be useful. It can show that something has accumulated, stabilized, drifted, plateaued, or changed. The issue is not whether weight matters. The issue is what kind of information it provides. Weight is evidence. It is not the explanation itself. Its meaning depends on the system pattern that produced it. A downstream signal becomes useful when it is read in relation to the upstream conditions that shape it. It can confirm that an outcome has emerged, but it cannot identify the cause on its own. Weight can show that a visible result has formed, but it cannot distinguish whether that result reflects intake pattern, expenditure shift, storage and release dynamics, fluid balance, recovery demand, appetite pressure, adaptation, compensation, or the accumulation of time. The number is therefore useful, but incomplete. It carries information, but not enough to stand alone.

Calling weight downstream protects interpretation from becoming too narrow. A number on a scale cannot reveal which upstream process changed, how long that change has been forming, or whether the current reading reflects fluid, glycogen, storage, recovery, digestion, or longer-term trend. It compresses many processes into one visible output. Compression creates visibility, but it also removes context. Without reconnecting that output to the processes that produced it, interpretation becomes detached from the system it is meant to describe.

Long-term weight stability emerges from coordinated regulation. No single mechanism produces it alone. Intake matters, but intake enters a responsive system. Expenditure matters, but expenditure is distributed and adaptive. Storage and release matter, but they are normal buffering functions operating across time. Appetite matters, but it reflects regulatory pressure rather than character. Hormonal signaling matters, but signals coordinate the system rather than replacing it.

These mechanisms do not operate as separate departments. They overlap continuously. Intake influences storage and immediate availability. Storage influences what can be released later. Availability influences appetite pressure and perceived energy. Appetite shapes future intake exposure. Expenditure shifts with activity, recovery demand, and compensation. Recovery itself redistributes energy and fluid toward repair. Hormonal signaling coordinates routing among these domains, shaping how energy is used, stored, or released at different times.

Sleep, stress, and recovery conditions alter the environment in which all of these processes occur. Adaptation changes how the system responds to repeated conditions. Compensation adjusts variables when one part of the system changes. None of these operate in isolation. The system behaves as an integrated structure in which each process both influences and is influenced by others. Outcome stability emerges not from any single variable behaving correctly, but from the interaction among many variables producing a coherent result across time.

This book has focused on the visible outcome layer. Earlier books in the series has examined upstream systems—how fasting changes input timing, how glucose reflects energy availability, how electrolytes maintain signaling stability, how metabolic flexibility shapes transitions between fuel states. Those mechanisms describe how the system operates internally. This book addresses where many of those internal processes become visible in a compressed form.

Weight is often where the system becomes noticeable. It is one of the most accessible outputs of complex regulation. That accessibility gives it importance, but also creates the risk of misinterpretation. Because weight is visible, it is easy to treat it as the primary explanation rather than as the surface expression of deeper processes. The visible outcome layer must therefore be reconnected to the upstream system. Without that connection, the number appears more definitive than it is.

Weight becomes more useful when it is interpreted as delayed evidence. A number on a given day is not a verdict. It is not immediate feedback on character, effort, discipline, or correctness. It is a delayed output influenced by prior conditions. It may reflect what the system has been doing for days, weeks, or longer. The reading belongs to a timeline, not a single moment. Delayed evidence changes how the number is understood. It may reflect accumulated prior conditions rather than the most recent action. It may lag behind internal changes that have not yet become visible. It may move temporarily because of short-term variability rather than long-term direction. This delay makes immediate interpretation fragile, because the visible output does not align cleanly with the moment it is observed.

This is why time, trend, context, and pattern are essential. A point can be accurate and still be incomplete. A trend can reveal what isolated readings cannot. Context can explain why two similar numbers may represent different system states. Pattern can show whether the output is stable, drifting, rebalancing, or changing direction. Without these layers, the number is too easy to overread.

The number matters less than the system pattern producing it because identical numbers can come from different internal arrangements. Two people, or two periods within the same person, may show the same weight while differing in appetite pressure, glucose handling, recovery demand, fluid balance, stress load, movement, storage access, or adaptation. The visible output is the same, but the system state is not.

Different numbers can also arise from similar system behavior under different conditions. Fluid shifts, glycogen status, recovery demand, inflammation, or digestive contents can alter the visible output without representing a different long-term system pattern. The scale compresses information. Pattern restores context. Pattern reconnects the number to time. It shows whether readings are clustering within a range, drifting gradually, stabilizing after change, fluctuating with variability, or holding in a temporary equilibrium. It allows the observer to distinguish between signal and noise without assigning meaning to any single point.

Pattern also separates observation from judgment. When the number is viewed as part of a pattern, it becomes a piece of information rather than a standalone evaluation. The emphasis shifts from what the number "means" in isolation to how it fits within a longer sequence of outputs. This shift stabilizes interpretation by placing the number back into the system that produced it.

Outcome stability does not mean the number never moves. It means the visible output remains interpretable within a stable system pattern. Fluctuation can occur inside stability. Variation can occur without drift. A plateau can occur without failure. Slow movement can occur when accumulated conditions become visible. Stability is not the absence of motion; it is coherence across time. Coherence means the output can be understood in relation to the conditions producing it. A stable system may still show variation, but that variation fits within an interpretable range. A changing system may still be coherent if the change reflects accumulated conditions rather than random noise. Outcome stability is not stillness. It is the presence of an interpretable relationship between system behavior and visible output.

This makes outcome stability a relationship between the system and its output. The number is the visible layer. The system pattern is the explanatory layer. When the two are interpreted together, weight becomes more informative. When the number is isolated, interpretation becomes fragile.

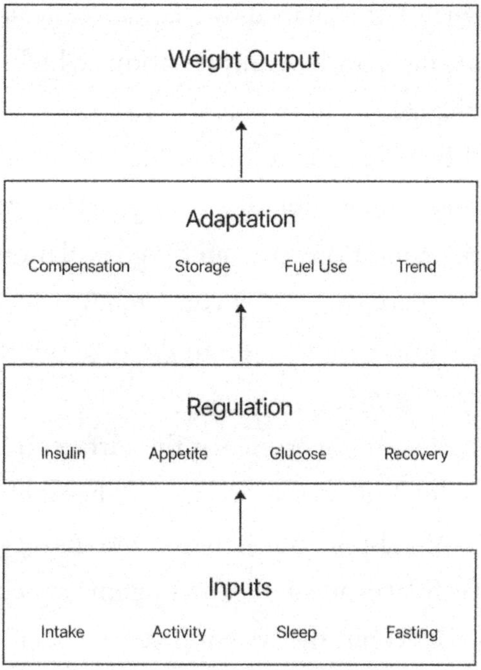

[Figure 16: System Pattern and Weight Output]

The figure represents weight as the visible output of coordinated upstream system behavior. Intake, expenditure, storage, release, appetite, hormonal signaling, glucose handling, fasting structure, flexibility, recovery, adaptation, compensation, trend, consistency, and time all contribute to the pattern that produces the number. The number is not the standalone cause or explanation.

The final body chapter returns to the frame that has structured the book. Weight is an output. It is shaped by lag, which separates input from visibility. It is shaped by variability, which introduces noise. It is shaped by intake and expenditure, which operate inside a responsive system. It is shaped by storage and release, which buffer energy across time. It is shaped by hormonal coordination and appetite, which regulate availability and demand. It is shaped by adaptation, which alters response to repeated conditions, and by compensation, which adjusts variables when conditions change.

It is also shaped by plateau and drift, which describe how the output behaves across time, and by glucose, fasting, and metabolic flexibility, which influence the conditions surrounding regulation. It is shaped by trend, which reveals pattern, and by consistency, which clarifies signal. Each of these mechanisms contributes to the structure that produces the visible number.

Weight stability, then, is not created at the surface. It emerges from the coordination of these processes across time. The number is where that coordination becomes visible, but it is not where it is determined. The visible output is the final expression of an ongoing system.

The number is visible, but the system pattern gives it meaning. Weight stability emerges from coordinated regulation across time, not from a single reading or isolated mechanism. The number matters less than the system pattern producing it.

Stability Before Control

Weight is visible, measurable, and easy to isolate. It appears as a number that can be recorded, compared, and followed across time. That visibility gives it an unusual authority. It feels immediate and definitive, as though it should explain itself. But throughout this book, a different frame has been established. Weight is not the system. It is an output produced by a system that operates through delay, variability, regulation, buffering, adaptation, compensation, and accumulation across time.

Returning to that frame at the end of the book clarifies what the number can and cannot do. Weight can show that something has occurred. It can show that conditions have accumulated into a visible outcome. But it cannot, on its own, explain what produced that outcome. The number is the surface of a deeper structure. It reflects the system without revealing it directly.

This is why control is the wrong starting point for interpretation. Weight is often approached as something that should respond directly and immediately to input changes. The expectation is that a change in intake or activity should produce a clear and proportional change in output. When that does not occur, the result can appear inconsistent or difficult to explain. The issue is not that the system is unpredictable. The issue is that the frame is too narrow.

The body does not operate like a simple control panel. Inputs do not pass through unchanged into outputs. They are received, interpreted, and distributed across a system that must maintain function while responding to changing conditions. Energy is routed, stored, released, and buffered. Appetite adjusts. Expenditure shifts. Recovery demands change. Hormonal signals coordinate timing and allocation. Adaptation alters future response. Compensation modifies variables when conditions shift. All of this unfolds across time before the output becomes visible.

Within that structure, control is not absent, but it is indirect. It does not begin at the level of the number. It begins with the conditions that shape the system. When control is treated as the starting point, interpretation collapses too quickly onto the output. When stability is treated as the starting point, the system remains visible.

Stability provides a broader and more durable frame. It directs attention to the conditions that produce the output rather than to the output alone. Stability does not require the number to remain fixed. It does not require the absence of variation. It refers to the coherence of the system across time—the way repeated patterns of intake, expenditure, storage, release, appetite, recovery, sleep, stress, and adaptation produce a visible outcome that can be understood in relation to those conditions.

A stable system may still fluctuate. It may show short-term variability, temporary plateaus, or gradual drift. These movements do not contradict stability. They occur within it. Stability is not stillness. It is the presence of an interpretable relationship between the system and its output. When that relationship is clear, the number becomes easier to understand. When it is unclear, the number becomes difficult to interpret, regardless of its value.

None of this requires weight to be ignored or dismissed. The number remains useful. It can reveal that change has occurred, that conditions have accumulated, that the system is maintaining a range or shifting over time. The problem is not the number itself. The problem is treating it as a complete explanation. When the number is separated from the system that produces it, it appears more decisive than it is. When it is placed back inside that system, its meaning becomes more accurate.

Weight is best understood as delayed evidence. A reading on a given day does not belong entirely to that day. It reflects prior conditions—patterns of intake, expenditure, recovery, stress, sleep, and adaptation that have been accumulating before the measurement was taken. It may also reflect short-term factors such as fluid balance, glycogen status, digestion, or recovery demand. These influences can shift the visible output without representing a change in longer-term direction.

Because of this delay, immediate interpretation becomes fragile. A single reading may be accurate and still incomplete. It may show a momentary state rather than a sustained pattern. This is why time, trend, and context are necessary. A pattern across time reveals more than any isolated point. It shows whether the system is maintaining stability, drifting gradually, rebalancing after change, or moving in a new direction. The number becomes more meaningful when it is placed within that pattern.

Placing the number back inside the system that produces it is the central movement of this book. The system includes energy intake and expenditure, but it also includes storage and release, appetite regulation, hormonal coordination, glucose handling, fasting structure, metabolic flexibility, sleep, stress, recovery, adaptation, compensation, trend, consistency, and time. These processes do not operate separately. They interact continuously, shaping the conditions under which weight is produced.

The number compresses these processes into a single visible output. Compression allows the output to be observed easily, but it removes detail. Without reconnecting the number to the system, interpretation remains incomplete. With that connection restored, the number becomes part of a larger structure rather than a standalone signal.

A calmer interpretive model follows from this structure. The number does not need to be treated as a verdict. It does not need to carry immediate judgment. It does not need to explain the entire system in a single moment. It can be observed as a point within a pattern, as delayed evidence within a timeline, as an output shaped by conditions that extend beyond the present reading.

This does not remove uncertainty, but it reduces misinterpretation. Variability can be recognized as part of biological output rather than as contradiction. Plateaus can be understood as temporary equilibrium rather than as absence of activity. Drift can be seen as accumulated mismatch rather than sudden change. Trend can be used to distinguish pattern from noise. Consistency can clarify the relationship between conditions and output. Outcome stability can be understood as coherence across time rather than as stillness.

These shifts do not change the system. They change how the system is read. The same number can be interpreted in multiple ways depending on the frame applied to it. A narrow frame compresses meaning into the number itself. A broader frame restores the system that produced it.

This is where the title-level idea of the conclusion settles. Stability comes before control, not because control is impossible, but because control cannot be understood without first understanding the system that produces the output. The number is visible, but visibility is not explanation. Control language narrows interpretation to the surface. Stability language keeps the full structure in view.

Across the book, weight has been presented as an output shaped by lag, variability, intake, expenditure, storage, release, appetite, hormonal coordination, adaptation, compensation, plateau, drift, glucose signaling, fasting structure, metabolic flexibility, trend, consistency, and time. None of these mechanisms replaces the others. They interact. The output that appears on the scale is the result of that interaction across time.

The conclusion does not add a new mechanism. It returns to the central frame with greater clarity. Weight is not the system. It is the visible result of system behavior. Its meaning depends on how it is interpreted, and interpretation depends on whether the number is read in isolation or within the structure that produced it.

Understanding weight begins when the number is no longer mistaken for the system itself. It begins when the number is read as an output: delayed, variable, and shaped by many interacting conditions across time.

About the Author

Nathan Reed writes about metabolic stability in systems exposed to load, variability, and time.

His work examines how biological capacity is shaped by energy availability, recovery architecture, sleep amplitude, muscle mass, environmental demand and workload. Rather than treating nutrition, fasting, sleep, and training as isolated tactics, he approaches them as interacting regulatory systems governed by margin, buffering, oscillatory coherence, and constraint dominance.

The Stability framework explores how physiological compression accumulates gradually and how proportional calibration preserves long-horizon resilience across decades. The objective is not peak optimization, but preservation of functional continuity under load.

Weight Stability is part of a broader metabolic stability ecosystem developed under Perennial Publishing, each volume addressing a distinct vector of biological durability.

The work is designed for readers who prefer structural clarity over motivational rhetoric and long-horizon coherence over short-term intensity.

The Metabolic Stability Series

Metabolic Stability: *A Systems Guide to Blood Sugar, Fasting, and Long-Term Metabolic Health*

(Cornerstone Volume)

Fasting Fundamentals: *A Systems Guide to Metabolic Flexibility, Fat Loss, and Long-Term Health*

(Foundational Volume)

Intermittent Fasting: *Metabolic Timing, Body Composition, and Sustainable Health*

Prolonged Fasting: *A Systems Guide to Duration, Recovery, and Metabolic Limits*

Electrolytes: *A Systems Guide to Hydration, Electrolyte Balance, and Physiological Stability*

Insulin Stability: *Blood Sugar, Insulin Resistance, and Metabolic Health*

Glucose Stability: *How Blood Sugar Fluctuations Affect Energy, Insulin, and Metabolic Health*

Metabolic Flexibility: *How the Body Switches Between Fat and Glucose for Energy and Metabolic Health*

Future Titles Include:

Energy Stability

Adaptation and Drift

The Vitality Series:

Sleep and Recovery

Strength and Aging

Hormones & Sexual Health

Part of a Broader Stability Framework

The Metabolic Stability Series is part of a larger stability ecosystem published by Perennial Publishing.

Related domains include:

Money Stability — structural durability in financial systems

Career Stability — positioning, load tolerance, and transition resilience

Mental Stability — cognitive steadiness under pressure and uncertainty

Emotional Stability — regulatory steadiness in environments that do not slow down

Foundations — low-fragility life architecture

Vitality — energy, strength, and biological function across time

Each domain approaches stability as a structural problem: capacity versus load, buffering versus shock, governance versus drift. Together, they form a unified framework for long-horizon durability across the major systems that shape human trajectory.

About Perennial Publishing

Perennial Publishing produces practical systems guides for building stability in an unstable world.

Our books explore the foundations of long-term resilience across health, finance, career, and everyday decision-making. Each title focuses on clear frameworks, durable principles, and practical strategies that help readers build lasting stability rather than short-term fixes.

The Perennial catalog includes series on metabolic health, financial stability, career systems, and personal consistency. While each book stands on its own, they share a common goal: helping individuals create durable systems that support a stable and sustainable life.

Made in the USA
Monee, IL
05 November 2026

67386763R00083